the**facts**

Sleep problems in children and adolescents

➲ also available in the**facts** series

thefacts

Sleep problems in children and adolescents

PROFESSOR GREGORY STORES

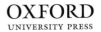
OXFORD
UNIVERSITY PRESS

OXFORD

UNIVERSITY PRESS

Great Clarendon Street, Oxford OX2 6DP

Oxford University Press is a department of the University of Oxford.
It furthers the University's objective of excellence in research, scholarship,
and education by publishing worldwide in

Oxford New York

Auckland Cape Town Dar es Salaam Hong Kong Karachi
Kuala Lumpur Madrid Melbourne Mexico City Nairobi
New Delhi Shanghai Taipei Toronto

With offices in

Argentina Austria Brazil Chile Czech Republic France Greece
Guatemala Hungary Italy Japan Poland Portugal Singapore
South Korea Switzerland Thailand Turkey Ukraine Vietnam

Oxford is a registered trade mark of Oxford University Press
in the UK and in certain other countries

Published in the United States
by Oxford University Press Inc., New York

© Oxford University Press, 2009

British Library Cataloguing in Publication Data

Data available

Library of Congress Cataloging in Publication Data

Stores, Gregory.
  Sleep problems in children and adolescents: the facts / Gregory Stores.
    p. cm.—(the facts)
  Includes index.
  ISBN 978–0–19–929614–9
  1. Sleep disorders in children—Popular works. 2. Sleep disorders in adolescence—Popular
works. I. Title
  RJ506.S55S76 2009
  618.92'8498—dc22

                                                                    2008033835

ISBN 978–0–19–929614–9

10 9 8 7 6 5 4 3 2 1

Typeset in Plantin
by Cepha Imaging Pvt. Ltd., Bangalore, India
Printed in China through
Asia Pacific Offset

Foreword

In almost all human societies, folklore and mythology are filled with stories of the consequences of inadequate or excessive sleep. In the 16th century, Thomas Phaire, arguably one of the first British paediatricians, recognized many of the disturbances of sleep in childhood and their implications for the family. Despite this wide-spread cultural recognition of the importance of sleep and sleep disorders in childhood, such disorders have, to a large extent, been ignored for many years by orthodox medical practitioners. This lack of awareness and understanding of the potential importance of sleep disorders is exemplified by the fact that the current edition of a widely used international textbook of paediatrics contains just five pages on children's sleep disorders out of a total of 2,600.

Recent developments in our understanding brought an appreciation of the importance of sleep problems in childhood and their potential consequences in later life very much to the fore of medical research as the long-term consequences of inadequate or insufficient sleep during mid- to late-childhood (including obesity and high blood pressure) have been increasingly recognized.

In this extremely valuable book, Professor Stores sets out in language that is accessible to those without a scientific or technical background what is known and what can be done in the complex, rapidly expanding field of children's sleep disorders. This book will, I am certain, be of immense value to parents, to teachers, and to those working with children in a wide range of settings. I am sure it will also be of enormous help to many healthcare professionals (including paediatricians) who wish to understand the implications and importance of normal sleep patterns, how they are vulnerable to disruption and how they can be protected during the crucial years of childhood and adolescence.

Sleep, like nutrition and physical activity, is an area of human activity far too important to be left to the professionals and this book, in helping to raise public awareness and knowledge of what is known in this field, will, I believe, be of considerable value, both directly and indirectly, to children and young people.

Peter J. Fleming
Professor of Infant Health and Developmental Physiology

Preface

Sleep problems in children and adolescents are very common and are often the cause of concern and distress for both the child and the family. They can affect behaviour, learning, and sometimes physical health. As there are many possible causes of these problems (some psychological, others physical), it is essential to identify the one responsible in your own child, because this will show what advice or treatment is needed.

The book starts by explaining the importance and nature of sleep and the changes that occur as your child grows up. How to recognize that your child's sleep is unsatisfactory is explained. The book then describes why children may not sleep well at different ages from babyhood to adolescence, the causes of excessive sleepiness during the day, and types of unusual behaviour or experiences that a child can have at night. The various types of treatment needed for these problems are described. The later chapters discuss those children who are especially liable to have sleep problems, the ways in which such problems may be mistaken for other conditions, the means by which unsatisfactory sleep can be spotted at home and at school, and how to get help for your child's sleep problem. Throughout the book, cases are described to illustrate how various sleep disorders can be correctly diagnosed and treated.

The book is intended to raise awareness of the importance of children's sleep disorders, as well as their recognition and treatment. It is written mainly for parents, but will also be of interest to anyone involved in the care and welfare of children.

Professor Gregory Stores
April 2008

Contents

Introduction

> **❌ Myth versus fact**
>
> **Myth:** Very little is known about sleep.
>
> **Fact:** This is definitely not true. Much has been discovered scientifically about sleep and its disorders in people of all ages. The problem is that this knowledge is not known to the general public and many professionals, with the result that many opportunities are missed for helping people with sleep problems.

It must be the case that from earliest times children have caused their parents grief because they would not or could not sleep well. Some early depictions of domestic scenes show babies sleeping contentedly, but quite the opposite is acknowledged in, for example, Thomas Phaire's *Boke of Chyldren*, the first paediatrics textbook in English, published in 1545.

Phaire's purpose in writing his book was to describe illnesses or disorders that he thought were particularly common in children, with recommendations for their treatment. In keeping with medical standards of the time, his remedies were highly imaginative. Quite how such notions were derived and their effectiveness are left fascinatingly obscure.

Among his list of 39 paediatric maladies, starting with '*apostume (swelling or abscess) of the brayn*' and ending with '*gogle eyes*' (squint), four sleep problems are discussed: '*watchying out of measure*' (sleeplessness), '*terryble dreames and feare in the slepe*' (nightmares), '*colyke and rumblying in the guttes*' (a potential cause of difficulty settling to sleep) and '*pyssing in the bedde*', now more prosaically called bedwetting or nocturnal enuresis.

As an example of Phaire's recommended treatments, for bedwetting he suggested the administration of powders made from the windpipe of a cock or the testicles of a hedgehog!

Curious though all this might sound, Phaire's attention to the special problems of children's sleep was unusual and remained so until fairly recently. An interesting and rare example in the literature was Dickens's description of Fat Boy Joe in *The Pickwick Papers*, which is so detailed that it is likely to have been based on a real person. Joe's excessive sleepiness is thought likely to have been the result of obstructive sleep apnoea, which will be discussed later.

Sporadic entreaties by professionals to take children's sleep problems seriously include the description in 1892 by the famous physician Sir William Osler of the psychological and physical effects of childhood obstructive sleep apnoea, warnings by Clement Dukes, a school doctor, in 1905 of both mental and bodily consequences of sleep loss in young schoolchildren, and the plea in 1978 by Thomas Anders and colleagues at Stanford University to pay more attention to the difficulties of excessively sleepy children, a plea still not sufficiently heeded.

The aim of this book is to help to correct the persisting relative neglect of the wide range of sleep disorders in children of all ages, including adolescents. Only a general account is provided here. The recommended reading at the end of the book provides more details, including references to individual studies. Reference to 'he' or 'his', and not the female gender, is for the purpose of brevity only; the conditions described apply equally to both sexes.

This book is not a substitute for seeking medical or other professional advice if sleep problems are severe or have failed to respond to simple self-help measures by parents.

Part I

General aspects of sleep and sleep disorders

1

Normal sleep

 Key points

- Sleep is an essential part of existence, without which there are serious psychological and physical consequences.

- Sleep is a biologically complicated state controlled by complex brain mechanisms that are involved in going to sleep, waking up, and switching between two very different types of sleep.

- An internal biological clock controls our periods of being asleep and awake, and also changes the levels of alertness and sleepiness within each 24 hours.

- Fundamental changes in sleep occur during childhood and adolescence.

Myth versus fact

Myth: Sleep is just the shutting down of daytime activities.

Fact: There are complex brain processes involved in going to sleep and in switching from one type of sleep to another.

Myth: Sleep is just one state, the opposite of being awake.

Fact: There are two distinct types of sleep. A balance between the two is probably required, especially in children.

What is sleep?

The most fundamental aspect of sleep is that it is an essential part of your existence in the sense that without it you cannot survive. Animal experiments have showed that, if kept constantly awake for approximately 10 days, rats undergo a profound deterioration in their basic bodily processes such as temperature control and they die.

As described in detail in this book, lesser degrees of sleep loss (and also poor-quality or broken sleep) can have serious, unwelcome psychological and even physical effects. Without regular periods of rest, animals are unable to function properly in all sorts of ways. Indeed, even plants can show clear periods of rest alternating with activity, usually but not necessarily coinciding with whether it is night or day.

Another basic feature of sleep is that, in humans and related species, it has very distinctive characteristics compared with other states of relative inactivity. The brain activity of hibernating animals is generally depressed as part of an overall slowing down of bodily processes. The same is true when someone is in coma or unconscious (for example, under a general anaesthetic). Sleep is different in a number of ways. For example, you can be roused from sleep but, in particular, sleep shows specific patterns of brain and other physiological activity.

Human sleep also shows additional interesting differences compared with other animal species. The duration of sleep within each 24-hour period varies from about 3 hours in a horse to almost 20 hours in bats. An adult human being holds a mid-way position with an average of 7–8 hours. These differences are perhaps partly explained by differing vulnerability to attack by predators, although other possible explanations have been suggested.

Humans usually sleep at night in a bed; hamsters, as an example, also sleep in their beds but during the day rather than at night. Some animals, such as cattle and horses, can sleep standing upright; others, such as leopards, may sleep in a tree. Dolphins and some other sea-dwelling mammals, who need to be awake enough to breathe intermittently at the surface, sleep in one half of their brain at a time, switching from one hemisphere to the other at intervals of minutes to hours.

Roosting birds are able to sleep while maintaining their balance on a perch. Fish and reptiles also sleep or at least rest regularly in a way similar to sleep.

Why do we need to sleep?

Whichever way animals sleep, they need to do so, because the consequences can be serious if not dire. Sleep can also be seen as particularly important from the fact that adult human beings spend about one-third of their life asleep and children much more than this (see below). In fact, by early school age, the average child has spent more time asleep than eating, playing, exploring his environment, or interacting with others.

There has been much debate about the function of sleep, with many suggestions being made. Clearly, there is no single answer to this question. Sleep serves many different, related functions, the balance between them changing during the course of development and possibly varying from one species to another.

Different theories have emphasized mental and bodily restoration and recovery during sleep, or the laying down of memories in the brain so that learning from experience is possible. Others have suggested that dreaming is essential for the analysis of possibly deep-seated emotional problems and conflicts. On the physical side, growth, resistance to infection, and possibly the process of repair following injury or other damage to body tissues depend on adequate sleep.

What can be said with assurance is that, in humans, poor sleep is highly likely to cause potentially profound psychological and physical changes, which can be reversed if the sleep pattern is restored to normal. Unfortunately, these facts are not sufficiently well known by the general public and many professionals (including those involved in the health and welfare of children). Many parents are unaware that the sleep problems of their children can often be prevented or treated effectively, with the consequence that much unnecessary distress is caused both to the children and also to their parents.

Sleep is a biologically complex process

It might be thought that sleep consists mainly of the shutting down of daytime activities. This is certainly not the case. The onset of sleep, waking up, and the two distinct types of sleep all involve complicated biochemical changes in different parts of the brain.

Sleep is not just one state. In fact, there are two very different types of sleep: non-rapid eye movement (NREM) sleep and rapid eye movement (REM) sleep. The reason why there are two contrasting types is not clear. It seems that a balance between these two types is necessary to function well.

NREM sleep

In adults, this type makes up about 75% of sleep. It is divided into four levels of increasing depth, called stages, each of which has its own characteristic brain wave activity as recorded by an electroencephalogram or EEG. As sleep progressively deepens, increasing amounts of slow brain activity are seen.

Stages 1 and 2 are relatively light sleep; stages 3 and 4 are deep sleep from which it is particularly difficult to waken. Most deep sleep (which is also called slow wave sleep or SWS) occurs in the first 3 hours of overnight sleep. It is in this depth of sleep that sleepwalking and related disorders (see Chapter 15) occur. Fragments of dreams can occur in NREM sleep.

REM sleep

This is also called dreaming sleep because it is when most dreaming occurs. From the age of 2 and above, REM sleep comprises 25% of our sleep, but in newborns REM sleep takes up at least 50% of sleep (and more than this before birth). This suggests that it is particularly important for early brain development. It appears to play some part in memory although the details are unclear. In infants, the term 'active' sleep is used rather than REM sleep and at this age 'quiet' sleep is equivalent to NREM sleep.

At any age, the level of brain activity in REM sleep is high. For example, blood flow through the brain is increased compared with NREM sleep. EEG traces are similar to those recorded when you are awake and alert, yet it is not usually possible to move in this type of sleep, although some people can do so and, as a result, can act out their dreams (see Chapter 16). Another feature of REM sleep that is different from NREM sleep is prominent eye movements, and heart rate and breathing tend to be less regular in REM sleep.

It is possible that everyone dreams, but only some people can recall their dreams. Even blind people dream, although without any visual imagery if they have been blind from birth or from a very early age. Often, the content of dreams is a mixture of fragments of recent experiences or things that on your mind, but sometimes children and adults have recurrent upsetting dreams with a consistent theme based on distressing past experiences. Nightmares (see Chapter 16) are particularly frightening dreams; as they are related to REM sleep (which mainly occurs later in overnight sleep), they tend to occur later in the night. Dream-like experiences can occur when drifting off to sleep or in a drowsy state before waking up properly.

As illustrated in Figure 1.1, which shows the pattern of sleep stages in a healthy child, periods of NREM and REM sleep alternate with each other

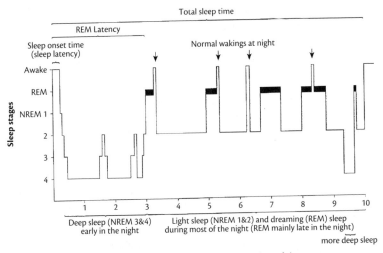

Figure 1.1 Hypnogram showing the characteristic progression of sleep stages overnight in a healthy school-aged child (from a book published by Mac Keith Press)

several times throughout the night. Ideally, a short while after settling into bed, drowsiness is followed by progressively deeper levels of NREM sleep. A period of deep NREM sleep, lasting 2–3 hours, is then followed by a brief first period of REM sleep. The rest of the night consists of alternating periods of light NREM sleep and increasingly long REM sleep periods, in children possibly ending with a more deep sleep before they finally wake up.

It is normal for anyone to wake briefly during the night, perhaps several times, although this may not be remembered. A problem only arises if it is difficult to get back to sleep at these times.

Complicated brain mechanisms control many of our bodily functions that fluctuate rhythmically:

♦ over a period of a day ('circadian' rhythms, such as our sleeping–waking cycle);

♦ over less than a day ('ultradian' rhythm, e.g. alertness fluctuations); and

♦ over more than a day ('infradian', e.g. the menstrual cycle).

When we sleep is regulated by a **circadian body clock** located in the supra-chiasmatic nucleus, which is part of the hypothalamus situated in the depths of the brain. This body clock usually ensures that the sleep–wake cycle is synchronized with the fluctuations in body temperature and the output of cortisol, a hormone involved in the response to stress. For example, body temperature falls during overnight sleep, being lowest in deep NREM sleep. Problems arise when these bodily processes become uncoupled as in jet lag or, more seriously, night-shift work. If this happens, sleep is disrupted and you are likely to feel uncomfortable or unwell in various ways.

From an early age, the sleep–wake cycle becomes linked with the night–day cycle by the influence of external cues ('zeitgebers'), the main one being the experience of daylight. Other cues are mealtimes and social activities, which become particularly important for blind people deprived of the main zeitgebers.

The suprachiasmatic nucleus is acted upon by **melatonin**, a hormone pro-duced mainly in the pineal gland in the brain during darkness ('the hormone of darkness') and suppressed by the perception of bright light. Therefore, mela-tonin promotes sleep during the night and its suppression by daylight encour-ages wakefulness. Synthetic melatonin has been used to treat some disorders of the sleep–wake cycle (see Chapter 7) including those caused by blindness.

The natural sleep–wake cycle lasts about 24 hours, but this can be disrupted by exposure to light while studying or working late at night. Lack of sleep will result from then having to get up in time for school, college, or work before sleep requirements have been met.

Alertness and the degree of sleepiness varies within each 24 hours. The tendency to sleep is greatest in the early hours of the morning at the time of deep NREM sleep. Trying to work at this time is difficult, and mistakes and accidents (including driving accidents) may well occur. To a lesser extent, sleepiness increases in the early afternoon (the 'post-lunch dip'). Use is made of this in countries where having a siesta is the rule.

Generally, we are most alert in the evening before the onset of sleepiness. This can be the best time to study. Parents should avoid putting their child to bed too early, i.e. during this period, because he will be unable to sleep, which is distinct from refusing to settle.

The timing of the different levels of alertness and sleepiness can be different from one person to another (including children). From an early age, some people wake up about 2 hours earlier than most other people and are very alert in the morning but then tire early in the evening. These are so-called 'morning types' or 'larks'. In contrast, others tend to wake relatively late and have difficulty getting going in the morning, but become alert and active in the evening, perhaps until quite late ('evening types' or 'owls').

Not surprisingly, larks have special difficulty coping with night-shift work because, in these people in particular, they are required to be active when their body clock is telling them to sleep.

These ultradian sleep–wake rhythms also vary at different ages. The body clock change that occurs at puberty is important in explaining the sleep problems that are particularly common in adolescents (see Chapter 7). At this stage of development, there is a tendency for the sleep phase to shift to a later time than at an earlier age. This causes difficulty getting to sleep and, as a result, insufficient sleep may well be obtained by the time it is necessary to get up for school, college, or work.

Incidentally, the opposite shift (i.e. to an earlier onset of sleep) occurs in old age. An early bedtime may well mean waking in the early hours because the amount of sleep required has been obtained by that time. This 'early morning waking' in older people should not be misinterpreted as a sign of depression in which early waking is associated with inadequate sleep. Something similar can happen in children who have habitually been put to bed particularly early and have soon gone to sleep, in which case their bedtime should gradually be delayed.

Changes in sleep patterns during childhood

Another example of the complicated nature of sleep is the striking change in sleep patterns during childhood. Most obvious is the amount of sleep needed for satisfactory function during the day. This is obvious from Table 1.1, which shows the average amount of sleep that is needed at different ages to function satisfactorily during the day. Some healthy children need more and others less than the amounts stated.

Studies of premature babies show that prolonged sleep (up to 20 hours a day) begins well before birth. Full-term babies sleep approximately 17 hours, with at least 50% taking the form of 'active' or REM-type sleep as described above. One result is that they tend to wake more often and readily than at an earlier age. Also, infants pass directly into REM sleep when they fall asleep.

Because their body clock has not developed properly, the sleep–wake pattern of young babies is so irregular that they have to be fed repeatedly during the night. However, this should not be necessary by about 6 months of age, at which time

Table 1.1 Average sleep requirements at different ages in childhood and adolescence

Age	Sleep requirement
Newborn, full-term baby	16–18 hours
1 year	14 hours
2 years	13 hours
4 years	11.5 hours
7 years	10.5
10 years	9 hours
Adolescence (after puberty)	9 hours (possibly more)
Late adolescence	8 hours

the baby should be biologically able to confine feeding to the daytime, allowing his parents to sleep themselves at night.

By the end of the first year, most children sleep about 15 hours a day and daytime naps (originally taking up perhaps half of the total sleep time) should have started to reduce significantly until by about 3–4 years of age they have stopped completely in most children.

Through the toddler stage and later childhood, the gradual reduction in total time asleep steadily reduces until in later childhood (before puberty) most children need about 10 hours of sleep each night. Sleep is particularly sound at this age.

As mentioned above, puberty marks a change in the function of the circadian body clock. At this adolescent stage, it becomes physiologically difficult to get to sleep until later than before. This, combined with late-night study or social activities, can easily lead to insufficient sleep. Teenagers usually need at least 9 hours of sleep, without which they are at risk of various problems (see Chapter 7).

2

Disturbed sleep

Key points

- Sleep problems are very common in children in general.

- Some groups are at particularly high risk of such problems, such as those with a learning disability or other kind of medical or psychological disorder.

- There are many ways in which consistently disturbed sleep can affect children, both psychologically and sometimes physically; their emotional state, behaviour, and learning are likely to be affected.

- Parents (and older children) need to be aware of the warning signs that a child's sleep is inadequate or of poor quality.

- To establish the true nature and cause of a sleep problem, systematic enquiries need to be made (starting with the family doctor or his team) about certain key aspects of the situation; in some cases, additional information will be required from special further investigations.

- There are many possible forms of treatment from which a choice can be made, depending on the nature of the sleep problem and its underlying cause.

Myth versus fact

Myth: Serious sleep difficulties (including loss of sleep by parents) are an inevitable part of having children, especially in the early years.

Fact: Good sleep habits can be encouraged from very early on in most children.

Myth: Drug treatment is the only form of treatment for sleep problems.

Fact: Actually, medication is rarely appropriate. Instead, depending on the cause of a child's sleep problem, a choice can be made from a range of treatments of various types that are now available.

Ways in which sleep can be disturbed: sleep problems and sleep disorders

For practical purposes, it is essential to distinguish between a sleep 'problem' and a sleep 'disorder'.

There are just three basic sleep problems or complaints that parents or children themselves might have:

♦ not sleeping well (or 'sleeplessness');

♦ being too sleepy (sometimes called 'hypersomnia');

♦ behaving in unusual ways or having strange experiences in relation to sleep (i.e. when going to sleep, during sleep, or on waking up). This group of sleep disturbances is called 'parasomnias'.

Of course, someone might have more than one sleep problem, and one sleep problem may cause another.

These sleep problems are not diagnoses or conditions in their own right, no more than is 'breathlessness' or 'pain'. In order for the correct advice or treatment to be determined, it is necessary to identify the *cause* of the problem—in the case of sleep, this means the underlying sleep disorder. The following parts of this book are concerned with possible explanations for the types of sleep problem that can occur in young people from infancy to adolescence.

How common are sleep problems in childhood and adolescents?

The simple answer to the above question is: very common. They are often the cause of much distress, which could be avoided if their cause was correctly identified and the appropriate help provided.

Estimates vary but, from early years to adolescence, at least 25–30% of children in general have a sleep disturbance that is considered by parents, or by the children themselves, to be significant. However, as will be described in detail later, the nature of the sleep problem varies significantly with age. Bedtime difficulties and problems with night waking are common up to about 3 years of age, sleep disorders including nightmares and sleepwalking feature more in older children, and many adolescents suffer from difficulty getting to sleep and, as a result, being sleepy during the day.

However common such problems are in children overall, there are certain groups of children in which sleeping difficulties occur even more frequently. Such 'high-risk' groups include:

- children with a learning disability;

- other neurological disorders including autism;

- psychiatric problems;

- various types of medical problem.

Some medical and psychiatric medications can interfere with sleep, causing either sleepiness or difficulty sleeping.

Effects on children of persistently not sleeping well

Emotional state and behaviour

It is common knowledge that tired children often become fractious if they are not able to settle to sleep. If kept awake, the behaviour of 'overtired' children can become very difficult to handle; they become irritable, distressed, and even aggressive, much to the exasperation of their parents and possibly the concern of brothers or sisters witnessing such events.

Generally, these are only occasional occurrences, but in some children such problems are frequent and seriously disrupt family life. At a later age, especially at adolescence, persistent loss of sleep can have a depressing effect and lead to problems at home and at school, which will be discussed in later chapters.

In adults, loss of sleep or disrupted sleep tends to cause a reduction in activity as the degree of sleepiness increases. As just described, the opposite can occur in young children, causing the types of behaviour described in children said to have attention-deficit hyperactivity disorder (ADHD), characterized by overactivity, impulsiveness, and poor concentration.

It is important to distinguish between the sleep problems of ADHD children, which are the result of difficult daytime behaviour extending to bedtime, and a subgroup of children whose initial problem is a sleep disturbance, which results in daytime ADHD symptoms. Treatment of this second group needs to be directed to the sleep disorder. If successful, this can be expected to improve daytime behaviour. Stimulant drugs are not appropriate in this subgroup and may make matters worse by increasing the sleeping difficulty.

Disturbed sleep can affect a child's emotional state and behaviour in various other ways. Bedtime can become a source of distress if associated with frightening thoughts or experiences that are associated with various sleep disorders described later, including night-time fears. In addition, a child's bedroom should not be used as a place of punishment. Obviously, it is important not to confuse emotional upset at bedtime with naughtiness.

Intellectual function and education

There is convincing evidence that insufficient sleep can cause impairment in concentration, memory, decision-making, and the general ability to learn. Performance in tasks requiring sustained attention is particularly affected, as well as those requiring abstract thinking or creativity. Similarly, motor skills and reaction times can be affected.

A number of studies in various countries have shown that school examination results are, not surprisingly, affected, with potentially long-term consequences such as not getting on higher education courses because of poor grades or failing to perform well at work if the sleep problem continues.

Physical effects

As the production of growth hormone is closely linked to deep non-rapid eye movement (NREM) sleep, if sleep is seriously disrupted from an early age, physical growth may be affected. Obstructive sleep apnoea or OSA (see Chapter 10) can disrupt sleep from about the age of 2, causing the child to 'fail to thrive' and be smaller for his age than he should be. This contrasts with OSA in adults, which is associated with being overweight.

A number of other physical problems are thought sometimes to be caused by severe sleep disturbance including a reduced ability to resist infection and possibly to heal properly following injury. Various other effects (including the onset of diabetes) and problems with raised blood pressure, as well as menstrual and pregnancy problems in females, have also been described in adults.

Effect on family and other social effects

If a child repeatedly does not sleep well, the effect on his parents and other children in the family can be serious because their own sleep is disturbed and also because this is likely to lead to tensions within the family as a whole.

There have been reports that relationships between a parent and child can be severely tested to the point of increased use of physical punishment in extreme cases. Parents may disagree with each other about ways of dealing with the child's refusal to go to sleep at the required time or the child's insistence on joining them in their own bed after waking during the night. In these circumstances, marital relationships may become seriously strained.

Such family difficulties will be made worse if one or other parent has other problems such as financial or employment difficulties, or if either is depressed. A poorly supported single parent is likely to be at particular risk, especially if there is more than one child with a sleep problem.

As a result of the changes in behaviour that can result from sleep disturbance, the affected child's interpersonal problems may extend beyond his family. Irritable, difficult, or otherwise disturbed behaviour is likely to affect friendships. Relationships with teachers can easily suffer, especially if they are unaware that the behavioural problems are the result of inadequate or otherwise disturbed sleep.

In view of all of these potential complications to the child's life, it is essential that all concerned realise that they are at least partly the result of sleep disturbance for which effective treatment can be provided in most instances.

Signs of unsatisfactory sleep

Many parents of young children with a sleep problem know all too well that a problem exists, especially in the case of settling difficulties at bedtime, troublesome night waking, or waking very early. However, the nature of the underlying sleep disorder may not be clear to them, if only because they are unaware of the various possibilities; these possibilities will be considered later.

Ideally, a child's sleep at night should be long enough (in keeping with his age; see Chapter 1) and also of good enough quality to allow him to feel well and to function properly during the day. Good-quality sleep means sound, largely unbroken sleep including deep NREM sleep, which is thought to be the most restorative type of sleep. It is not a problem if a child needs rather less than the average for his age, provided he is not sleepy or affected in some other way during the day.

It is clear from the above discussions that the signs of unsatisfactory sleep go beyond simply the number of hours actually spent asleep each night. Indeed, parents may not have an accurate idea of even this measure, especially in older children and adolescents.

Parents should suspect that their child's sleep is not what it should be if he:

- always has great difficulty waking up in the morning (and possibly is particularly irritable at being woken);

- does not want to go to school or college because he is too tired;

- is said by his teacher to always be tired (especially wanting to have a nap at school);

- shows signs that his schoolwork or his behaviour has deteriorated for no obvious reason, or that he has lost interest in various activities such as sports or meeting friends;

- falls asleep doing his homework in the evening;

- wants a lot of caffeine-containing drinks;

- sleeps in very late at weekends;

- feels and generally behaves better after a good night's sleep.

By initiating a conversation (probably for the first time) with their child about his sleep pattern, parents may well get a new insight into nature and extent of the problem and the need for professional advice about how the problem should be tackled.

Assessment of sleep problems

The point has already been emphasized that it is essential in assessing someone's sleep problem to discover the underlying cause (or sleep disorder).

There are many possible ways of doing this, the choice depending on how complicated the problem seems to be.

Sleep history

From reading this book, for example, parents and even teenagers themselves can learn what basic aspects of the situation need to be identified to get an idea of the nature and possible cause of the sleep problem. However, the first port of call in obtaining professional advice would usually be the family doctor (or in the case of young children, the health visitor). Normally, they would take a 'sleep history' covering at least the following points:

◆ What exactly is your child's sleep problem?

◆ When did it begin and what has happened about it since?

◆ Has it been linked with any other problems in your child's development (such as illness, emotional upset, or disability), or with difficulties or changes in the family?

◆ How have you tried to deal with the problem so far?

◆ Have you had any professional help? If so, exactly what was it and did it work?

◆ In what ways has the sleep problem affected the family?

◆ Has anyone else in the family had a sleep problem and, if so, what type? Did they grow out of it?

The sleep history should also cover your child's overall sleep habits, including bedtime and waking-up time, and their sleeping environment, as well as daily activities in general. Table 2.1 outlines step by step the information about your child's typical 24-hour sleep–wake cycle that you need to know (as far as possible) so that his sleep problem can be defined and a start made on determining its underlying cause.

Parents are the main sources of information, as well as older children themselves, but siblings, teachers, and possibly other people may have made important observations. All these aspects, and possibly more, will be gone into in more detail if it is thought advisable to refer your child to a paediatric, psychiatric, or specialized sleep disorders clinic.

Table 2.1 Outline review of 24-hour sleep–wake pattern (modified according to child's age)

Time of day	Behaviour pattern
Evening	Time of evening meal
	Other evening activities
Bedtime	Preparation for bed. With whom?
	Time of going to bed
	Problems in going to bed
	Fears or rituals
	Wanting to sleep with someone else or other comforts
	Time taken to fall asleep
	Experiences when falling asleep
During the night	Waking: frequency and cause, and ability to go back to sleep
	Other episodes: their exact nature, timing, and frequency
	Other behaviours during sleep, e.g. snoring, bedwetting, restlessness
	The reactions of you and your partner to these night-time events
Morning	Wakes up on his own or needs waking up
	Difficulty waking up
	Time he finally wakes up
	Time he gets up
	Total duration of night's sleep
	Longest period of uninterrupted sleep
	On waking up: mood, feeling refreshed or not, any other experiences
Daytime	Sleepiness: details of naps in young children, or falling asleep at a later age
	Lethargy
	Difficult behaviour
	Depression
	Concentration and performance
	Other unusual episodes

Sleep diary

It can be helpful to keep a sleep diary every day (see example in Table 2.2) for 2 weeks as part of the initial assessment. This can provide useful information

Table 2.2 Example of a page from a sleep diary

Date	Sunday April 12
Time woke(n) up	9.20 a.m. (woken by mum)
Time got up	9.45 a.m. (hurried by mum)
What did he do between waking and getting up?	Lay quietly listening to radio. Seemed very tired.
Time/length of any daytime naps	Fell asleep after lunch (about 2.30 p.m.). Woken by sister at 3.30 p.m.
What was his behaviour like during the day?	Tended to be irritable and offhand.
What did he do in the hour before bedtime?	Played a computer game with sister, then watched TV. Reluctantly had a bath and complained he wasn't tired but eventually went to bed when prompted repeatedly.
Time to bed	9.30 p.m.
Time to sleep	Between midnight and 12.30 a.m.
What happened in between going to sleep and falling asleep?	Jimmy read for at least an hour, then listened to the radio before getting up briefly at about 11.30 p.m. for a drink. The next morning, he said he had been kept awake worrying about a maths test at school the next day.
Time and length of all wakes during the night. Please describe exactly what happened.	Woke up at about 3.30 a.m. to visit toilet, but went straight back to bed and was asleep within a few minutes.

about basic aspects of your child's general patterns of sleep and wakefulness, as well as various factors that might affect his sleep.

Questionnaires

Another useful record of the basics of the sleep problem and possible cause is a sleep questionnaire provided by the doctor, which you can complete for your child or at least parts of which can be filled in by your child if old enough.

Some questionnaires ask about sleep problems in general, whilst others concentrate on particular aspects such as breathing problems in sleep or the degree of sleepiness. Some are meant specifically for adolescents. The choice of questionnaire depends on the likely nature of the sleep disorder or, of course, your child's age.

It can be helpful for a sleep questionnaire to be completed before your child attends a clinic to show where the emphasis should lie when a detailed sleep history is taken. The results can be compared with those following treatment of the sleep disorder.

Wider aspects of history taking

In situations where more detail is needed (for example, if your child attends a hospital clinic), information about the following aspects may be very relevant for clarifying the problem and deciding treatment:

◆ your child's general physical and psychological development;

◆ illnesses or disabilities including past and current treatments;

◆ any psychiatric problems;

◆ the family situation including any problems such as your own mental health;

◆ whether other members of the family have had a sleep disorder (for example, sleepwalking often runs in families).

Physical and mental state examination

In situations where it seems that a medical disorder might underlie your child's sleep problem, he will need to be examined physically. For example, enlarged tonsils and adenoids is the most usual cause of breathing difficulties in sleep (obstructive sleep apnoea; see Chapter 10). Depending on the initial findings, more detailed investigations may require a specialist.

Similarly, assessment of your child's behaviour and their relationship with yourself (if only in a preliminary way initially) may suggest the nature and origin of some sleep problems. In complicated family situations, referral to a child psychiatrist or clinical psychologist might be appropriate.

Other hospital investigations

The assessments already described are usually sufficient to clarify the problem and determine what help is required, but in a proportion of cases, special sleep recordings are required, depending on the nature of the problem.

Polysomnography (PSG) consists of recording brain activity and other physical measures, mainly during overnight sleep. This is usually done in a hospital in a special room, although in some cases, depending on the type of recording needed, the recording can be done at home using a miniature portable device.

PSG involves the attachment of small button-like electrodes to the scalp, the side of the eyes (to record eye movement) and under the chin (to record muscle activity). This procedure (which is painless) allows the type of overnight sleep pattern shown in Figure 1.1 to be determined. Depending on what sleep disorder is suspected, other measurements (of breathing, for example, if OSA is suspected) can be included in the recording.

PSG can be continued during the day in order to measure just how sleepy your child is. This is done by means of a multiple sleep latency test (MSLT) where the child is allowed to fall asleep in a quiet room five times during the day. Sleepiness is measured by how long it takes him to fall asleep each time. In some conditions, such as narcolepsy (see Chapter 11), the results will also show a tendency to enter rapid eye movement or REM sleep much sooner than is usual.

If the nature of episodes of disturbed behaviour at night is unclear, it can also be useful to carry out audio/video recordings as well as PSG at night. Sometimes, this will show important features that have not been noticed previously. A simple recording taken by parents using a home recording system can be valuable in this way, providing the episodes are captured on tape.

If all that needs to be clarified is the overall timing of being asleep or awake (rather than the details of which type of sleep has occurred), actometry (also called actigraphy) can be used. This entails wearing a small recorder (actometer) like a wrist-watch, which measures body movements during the day and also at night when, if you are asleep, you do not move much. An example of a wrist actometer is shown in Figure 2.1, with a typical actometry readout shown in Figure 2.2.

Occasionally, it is appropriate to carry out blood or urine tests in an attempt to find out the cause of a child's sleep problem.

Treatment approaches

A common mistaken assumption that there is not much that can be done about sleep problems in either children or adults, and that, if treatment is available, it mainly takes the form of sleeping pills or medicine.

In fact, many forms of treatment for sleep disorders are now recognized and often have been shown to be effective. This makes it all the more unfortunate that

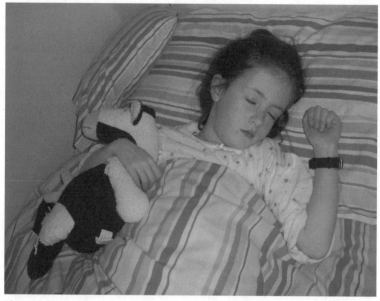

Figure 2.1 Example of the wristwatch like device used for actometry measurements.

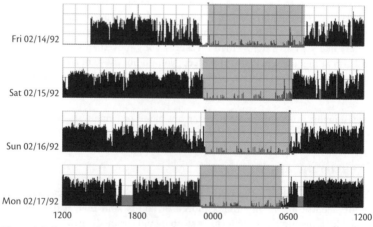

Fri 02/14/92

Sat 02/15/92

Sun 02/16/92

Mon 02/17/92

1200   1800   0000   0600   1200

Figure 2.2 Example of a continuous 96 hour actometer printout. Relatively little body movement occurred during periods of sleep. Reproduced with permission from Lucinda Wiggs.

relatively few of the many people troubled by disturbed sleep (either their children's or their own) do not ask for or receive the help available. Parents often believe that it is unavoidable that their children's sleep will be a problem (perhaps a serious problem) and that they have to put up with the consequences. As discussed later, this is not so.

The range of appropriate treatments is wide, with medication being justified in only very limited circumstances. The various treatments will be considered in detail later in relation to specific sleep disorders. Table 2.3 outlines the range of treatment approaches from which a choice should be made for the individual child, depending on his accurately defined sleep disorder.

General points

Giving parents an explanation of the nature and cause of the problem can itself be very therapeutic, especially if they have previously obtained confusing advice from various sources. Striking an optimistic note about treatment prospects is likely to be very comforting.

Reassurance can often be given about many forms of childhood sleep disorder. For example, arousal disorders such as sleepwalking (see Chapter 15) are likely

Table 2.3 Main advice and treatments for children's sleep disorders

	Treatment
General principles	Explanation, reassurance where appropriate, support
	Good sleep hygiene
	Safety or protective measures (e.g. in hazardous parasomnias)
	Treatment of any underlying medical or psychological disorder (but consider possible unhelpful effects of prescribed medication)
Specific measures	Behavioural (mainly for sleeplessness)
	Chronotherapy (for circadian sleep–wake cycle disorders)
	Medication (rarely hypnotic drugs; possibly melatonin especially for sleep–wake cycle disorders; stimulant drugs e.g. for narcolepsy; 'antidepressants' e.g. for parts of the narcolepsy syndrome)
	Physical procedures (surgery or continuous positive airway pressure for OSA)
	Psychiatric treatment where needed

to improve spontaneously in time. Even dramatic parasomnias very rarely indicate psychiatric disturbance.

Parental advice is important, for example to employ safety measures to lessen the risk of accidental injury in sleepwalking or headbanging (see Chapter13).

Bedtime settling problems and night-waking difficulties can be effectively treated by psychological methods (see Chapter 5), sometimes with surprisingly quick results, even in long-standing cases. Similar approaches can also be valuable in other childhood sleep disorders including severe nightmare problems.

In sleeplessness and excessive sleepiness due to mistiming of the sleep phase (common in adolescents; see Chapter 7), alteration of the timing by various means (chronotherapy) is required.

As already mentioned, medication for sleeplessness is rarely the answer because it is ineffective and can cause other problems. Melatonin has been used for sleeplessness but without justification in many cases. On the other hand, stimulant drugs have an important part to play in excessive sleepiness such as that caused by narcolepsy (see Chapter 11).

Physical measures may be needed, such as the removal of tonsils or adenoids and other ways of improving breathing during sleep in children with OSA (see Chapter 10).

Sleep hygiene

'Good sleep hygiene' deserves special mention. It refers to ways of promoting satisfactory sleep in anyone, whether or not you have a sleep disorder. For people with a sleep disorder, sleep hygiene principles can be combined usefully with more specific treatments.

The basic principles of good sleep hygiene for children and adolescents are outlined in Table 2.4. Their appropriateness varies with age. Several are particularly relevant to older children or adolescents who complain about awake lying in bed for long periods unable to sleep. It is important that bed does not come to be associated with difficulty sleeping. If someone does not fall asleep after about 20 minutes, it is better for them to move to another room for a while until they become tired enough to sleep.

Table 2.4 Basic principles of sleep hygiene (relevance varies with age)

Principle	Routine
Sleeping environment conducive to sleep	Familiar setting
	Comfortable bed
	Correct temperature
	Darkened, quiet room
	Non-stimulating
	No negative associations (e.g. struggles with parents or punishment)
Encourage	Bedtime routines
	Consistent bedtimes and waking-up times (weekdays, weekends, holidays)
	Going to bed only when tired
	Thinking about problems and plans before going to bed
	Falling asleep without parents (for young children)
	Regular daily exercise, exposure to sunlight, and general fitness
Avoid	Too much time awake in bed (especially if distressed)
	Overexcitement near bedtime and use of the bedroom as a place of entertainment
	Excessive or late napping during the day
	Late evening exercise
	Caffeine-containing drinks late in the day
	Smoking and excessive alcohol
	Large meals late at night

Part II

Sleep problems and their underlying causes

How to use this section of the book

This section takes in turn the three basic sleep problems (sleeplessness, excessive sleepiness, and parasomnias) and describes their possible underlying causes (sleep disorders) in children of different ages from babies to adolescents.

The first step in deciding what is relevant to your child is to consider in what particular way his sleep is a problem and then read about the possible causes in a child of his age. It is important to realise that the sleep patterns of healthy children vary from one child to another and also that what might seem unusual does not necessarily mean that there is something wrong and in need of treatment.

Your own knowledge of children's sleep and your expectations, as well as your emotional state and other people's opinions (which might be mistaken), can all influence your view of the situation and your judgement about whether help is really needed or not. However, if you are really worried about your child's sleep, it is important to tell your doctor or health visitor, if only to be reassured.

3

Sleeplessness

> ## ➲ Key points
>
> **Questions to ask yourself to help clarify the nature and possible reason why your child does not sleep well**
>
> ◆ In what precise way does your child not sleep well? Is it problems at bedtime, troublesome waking during the night, waking up very early in the morning, or a combination of these things?
>
> ◆ How much sleep does he get and is this appropriate for his age (see Chapter 1)?
>
> ◆ Is he tired or upset in any way during the day?
>
> ◆ Is his bedroom likely to help him get off to sleep easily and then to sleep soundly?
>
> ◆ Does he have a consistent relaxing time leading up to bedtime so that he is then ready to sleep?
>
> ◆ Has he any medical or psychological conditions that might disturb his sleep?
>
> ◆ Did his sleep problems follow any distressing experience such as changing school, moving house, illness, or death in the family?
>
> ◆ How has your child's sleep problem affected you or other members of the family?
>
> ◆ Have you had any advice or treatment for his sleep problem? What happened?

Some of the key points in helping to explain why your child is not sleeping well are described in this chapter. The importance of these and the other points mentioned here will be explained in later sections of the book.

Specific questions to ask that will apply to different age groups are:

Babies

◆ How often do you get up to feed your baby at night? How old is he?

Toddlers and pre-school children (1–4 years)

◆ Is your child still napping a lot during the day or taking his last nap near bedtime so that he is not tired enough to sleep?

◆ Is his bedtime very early?

◆ Does he insist on having you with him in order to get to sleep?

◆ Does he go to sleep downstairs or somewhere different from where he wakes in the night?

◆ Do you give in to his delaying tactics at bedtime or his demands for you to be with him if he wakes in the night?

◆ Does your child readily settle to sleep (or go back to sleep easily in the night) with one person but not another? If so, this suggests that one of you is not setting appropriate limits or that this person's relationship with the child is unsatisfactory in some other way.

Middle childhood (school age up to puberty)

The last set of points should be considered as well as the following.

◆ Is your child's bedroom an exciting, entertaining place or is it somewhere to relax ready for sleep?

◆ Is he unable to settle to sleep because he is afraid, rather than being naughty?

Adolescence

Again, some of the above questions should be asked but there are other possibilities, particularly at this age.

◆ As far as you can tell, is your child unable to get to sleep until it is very late?

- Is he particularly difficult to wake in the morning?

- Does he seem to be very sleepy during the day?

- Does he sleep in very late at weekends?

- Does you child seem worried or depressed?

- Does he drink a lot of coffee or other drinks that contain caffeine?

- Does he drink much alcohol or smoke?

- Do you suspect that he uses illegal substances?

> ## ❌ Myth versus fact
>
> **Myth:** Having a sleep problem simply means that you don't sleep well.
>
> **Fact:** There's a great deal more to it than that. There are different ways in which sleep can be disturbed and also many possible causes that need to be considered in both children and adults. The causes vary with age.

What does 'sleeplessness' mean?

Sleeplessness can mean one or more of the following:

- bedtime difficulties or 'settling problems' (either reluctance to go to bed or difficulty getting to sleep);

- waking up in the night and not being able to return to sleep without your attention or company;

- waking early in the morning, not going back to sleep again, and (usually) disturbing your own sleep or that of other people in the house.

Less often, 'sleeplessness' is used by parents in a different way to mean that their child's sleep is very restless or disturbed by frequent nightmares or other recurrent events at night. These different problems need to be distinguished, as their causes may well be different. Sometimes a child is, in fact, sleeping normally, but his parents' expectations are mistaken, causing them to worry unnecessarily. If this is the case, an explanation and reassurance may be helpful unless the parents are unable to take a balanced view because they are depressed or emotionally troubled in some other way.

How common are sleeplessness problems in children?

Sleeplessness (called 'insomnia' if the child is old enough to complain himself) is the main sleep problem in children. In infants and toddlers, sleep problems cause concern in about 25% of families. Perhaps 15% of older children mainly have settling problems and then the figure rises again to 20% or more of adolescents who have difficulties getting to sleep or staying asleep.

As mentioned previously, particularly high rates of sleeplessness and other sleep problems are seen in:

◆ children and adolescents with psychiatric problems;

◆ those with a learning difficulty or some other form of neurodevelopmental disorder such as autism; this can be caused by factors such as parents' difficulties handling their child, impairment of his ability to acquire good sleep habits, or an accompanying physical or psychiatric disorder;

◆ children with other chronic illness (e.g. those causing pain or breathing difficulties at night due to lung or heart disorders); this applies at any age.

Some forms of paediatric medication (such as those to help with breathing) may affect sleep. Also, admission to hospital, especially in intensive care, often causes sleep disturbances that can be persistent.

General points

Especially in their early years, most children need their parents' help in coping with night-time separation and the potentially frightening experience of the dark or their own thoughts and fantasies. Infants need the comfort of physical contact.

Children depend on their parents to provide positive attitudes to sleeping and the avoidance of negative associations such as arguments, punishment, and rejection.

Parents' ability to provide such help depends on their personality and sensitivity, their circumstances and mental state, and possibly also their attitudes to their child's sleep based on their own experiences in childhood.

An irregular sleep–wake pattern (i.e. disorganized and variable episodes of sleep) causes insomnia as well as daytime sleepiness. This can be just one aspect of a disorganized way of life that characterizes some families as a whole. Sometimes parents are not motivated to improve their child's sleep. For example, a child's presence in the parental bed might be welcomed by one partner as a means of distancing themselves from the other at night.

Drug treatment for sleeplessness is rarely justified. Conventional sleeping medicines for children (such as those containing antihistamines) are generally ineffective and may cause drowsiness or other problems during the day. The place of melatonin, which has sometimes been used for sleepless children, remains uncertain in view of the many unresolved issues surrounding its use.

As night-time and sleep onset may have particularly negative associations for psychologically disturbed children, special efforts may need to be made to help them make a smooth transition to restful sleep.

4

Babies who don't sleep well

Importance of babies' sleep

Good sleep is of vital importance at any age. In babies, who have the greatest need for sleep, it is thought to promote development of the brain processes in evaluating new daytime experiences and the development of new skills. Babies' sleep is probably also important for energy restoration, physical growth, and the function of the immune system, as well as certain other basic bodily processes. In addition, behaviour and social development depend on obtaining satisfactory sleep without which the baby may be irritable, generally out of sorts, and not functioning well, in a similar way to older children or adults who are short of sound sleep.

Unfortunately, in antenatal and parenting classes, parents are often not taught about sleep and ways of preventing or dealing with their children's sleep problems. Also, professionals involved in child healthcare generally do not learn much about these topics in their training. As a result, many babies fail to acquire good sleep habits as early as they might, or bad sleep habits become established, which may persist into later life. Many parents themselves suffer needless sleep loss and distress as a result of their child not sleeping well.

The size of these problems is considerable—about a quarter of families are significantly affected by their young children's sleep problems. As mentioned earlier, many more families than this have difficulties if children of this age (or older) have a chronic physical illness, a psychiatric disorder, or serious developmental problems. It is worth emphasizing, however, that sleep problems can be treated effectively in many children with such disorders, as well as children whose development is otherwise normal.

Sleep problems in babies

The most common problem in newborn babies (who initially sleep on average about 16 hours) is that parents' own sleep is disturbed by the need to feed the baby repeatedly at night. Newborns have not yet developed their internal body clock, which, in all of us, controls the pattern of sleeping and waking in relation to whether it is night or day. For this reason, and also because most of their time asleep is spent in so-called active sleep (see Chapter 1) from which it is easy to wake up, they wake frequently (about every 2–4 hours), usually when they are hungry.

Gradually, the longest period of sleep increases, and by 6 months a baby's body clock is sufficiently developed for him to be able to confine feeding to daytime and sleeping to night-time. However, from the time that the body clock begins to develop (about 6 weeks), parents can help it to be set so that the baby's main sleep period coincides with their own preferred sleep time at night (see below).

It is important to encourage good sleep patterns and habits in babies from the start in order to avoid bad sleep habits later on, such as bedtime problems or difficulties during the night. Ways of doing this are also often valuable in correcting bad sleep habits that have already developed.

Ways in which babies (and their parents) can get a good night's sleep

Important ways of helping to set the body clock and of teaching a baby good sleep habits are as follows. These are general guidelines that are likely to be effective in most babies. Some babies learn good sleep habits more readily than others, and it is important that parents persist with these measures and do not give up too soon.

Try to establish a **24-hour routine** for your baby regarding the time of starting the day, feeding times, bathing, going out, and settling to sleep at night. This daily routine should be as consistent as circumstances allow, although inevitably some flexibility will be necessary.

A **bedtime routine** is important because it will signal to your baby that it is time to go to sleep soon. Before putting baby to bed at about the time that will later become the evening bedtime, 20–30 minutes can be spent doing the same things in the same order each time such as bathing or washing your baby, changing into nightclothes, feeding, a cuddle, pulling the curtains, and kissing and saying good night. Part of this routine can be used when putting your baby down to sleep during the day or at other times of the night. A definite end-point to the routine will become associated with falling asleep.

Some babies benefit from being given a feed at the same time late in the evening (even if this means waking them up) in order to 'top them up' so that they sleep longer rather than wake up sooner because they are hungry. On the other hand, it can be helpful with some babies to reduce the amount of this last feed somewhat to lessen the chance of wet nappies and discomfort in the night.

Babies should be helped to **learn how to fall asleep alone**. If a baby can do this at bedtime, it will help him to go back to sleep after waking during the night. This is called 'self-soothing'. Waking up every so often is entirely normal at any age; a problem only arises if your baby becomes distressed because of an inability to get back to sleep.

To help your baby to become self-soothing, it is best to always put him into his cot when awake or drowsy, give him a kiss, say goodnight, and then leave him to go to sleep alone. If he cries, wait a few minutes rather than responding immediately, because some babies cry as they are falling asleep. The same applies during the night—crying does not necessarily mean that your baby is hungry and, given a little time, he may well settle back to sleep. If your baby falls asleep during a night-time feed, it may be necessary to try and gently keep him awake during the feed or to wake him up before settling him back into his cot.

As a further way of helping your baby to go to go to sleep or back to sleep on his own, **the circumstances in which he falls asleep should be the same in other respects as those he experiences when he wakes during the night**. Your baby should not fall asleep downstairs or in other circumstances or surroundings different from those that he will experience when he wakes in the night.

Although there can be no hard and fast rules because parents differ from one family to another in their preferences, having your baby in your own bed ('co-sleeping') if he cries during the night is not advisable because it impairs your baby's ability to become self-soothing, apart from the risk that his breathing may become obstructed (see safety measures below).

Night-time feeds should not be continued beyond the age when the body clock is developed sufficiently that they are no longer necessary—usually about 6 months of age in babies born at full term. Feeding beyond this point (and feeding very frequently at night every time the baby cries, which, as mentioned already, does not necessarily mean that he is hungry) can get in the way of establishing good sleep patterns. Apart from anything else, frequent feeds can lead to the intake of large amounts of fluid resulting in uncomfortable, wet nappies. The main clue that this is the reason for repeated night waking in babies older than approximately 6 months old is that they only return to sleep when they have been fed. The solution is gradually to reduce and then stop the night-time feeds. This can be effective in as short a time as 2 weeks or so.

From an early age, it is advisable to try and establish a **clear difference between day and night** to help develop your baby's body clock. He needs to learn that at night it is quiet, dark (light has a large effect on the body clock), and calm, and that it is not a time for interacting with others. This can be achieved by keeping light levels low, being quiet and calm, and not playing with your baby (in fact, keeping contact with him to a minimum). By contrast, when it is time to get up in the morning, light should be let into the room and activities generally increased, including washing and dressing, as well as feeding and playing.

Your **baby's sleeping environment** should overall be conducive to sleep, i.e. the right temperature and not noisy or well lit. It is also important that your the baby is kept comfortable during the night by avoiding wet nappies or other forms of discomfort.

These various practical measures, by themselves, will not be effective in babies (or, indeed, older children) if they have a **physical disorder** such as cow's milk allergy or a painful ear infection. Both of these conditions are likely to cause inconsolable crying and general distress that is not necessarily confined to one time of day and which may well be accompanied by other signs of physical illness such as fever in the case of infection.

So-called infantile colic occurs in otherwise healthy infants who, from about 2–3 weeks of age, cry inconsolably, including in the evening when they cannot settle to sleep. Traditionally, this has been thought to be the result of abdominal pain for which antispasmodic medication has been prescribed. However, there are now doubts about this interpretation and the value of such treatment, and some believe that such infants represent the upper range of babies' tendency to cry. In truth, the cause of the condition remains a mystery. Typically, the problem seems to resolve by about 3 months of age, although sleep problems may continue if bedtime has become associated with both the child and parents being distressed.

Case study

Night-time feeding problems

A happy and healthy 12-month-old baby boy settled easily to sleep after a feed at about 7 p.m. but was still waking up to be fed every 2–3 hours throughout the night. This meant his parents' evening was disrupted, but, more seriously, his mother had to get up frequently in the night in order to bottle-feed him and change his wet nappy. This had been the situation since birth, and his mother had decided that, to avoid her husband being tired at work, she alone should give her baby his night-time feeds. As she was inevitably extremely tired during the day, she had become increasingly impatient with his night-time demands on her.

His mother asked the advice of her health visitor, who reassured her that, at his age, her baby was not actually hungry despite all the feeds she was giving him. It was simply a matter of habit that he cried for a feed each time he woke up, because feeding had become associated with going to sleep rather than signalling real hunger in the night.

It was recommended that a bedtime routine should be started that included feeding but involved him being settled whilst still awake. Then, when he initially awoke in the night, his mother was advised to go to him but for a much shorter time than before and with no eye or verbal contact. She was also told to provide a progressively weaker milk concentration until eventually he had only water towards the end of the night.

His parents very quickly established the bedtime settling routine. There was some crying initially, but within a few days this had stopped. Reducing the night-time feeds in the way recommended produced an almost immediate positive response. After about a week, he was settling well and sleeping throughout the night.

Safety measures

In addition to tips about teaching babies good sleep habits, advice is available about safety measures that all parents should practice to reduce the risk of their baby coming to harm during the night. These are concerned mainly with ensuring that the baby can breathe properly when asleep. The following are the main important points. Further details should be available from a health visitor or someone else with special experience of how to ensure babies' safety at night.

- Place your baby on his back in the cot.

- Use a good-quality, firm mattress, not a surface that can be compressed or moulded around your baby's face.

- Use a safety-approved cot with narrow gaps between the rails.

- Your baby's face and head should not be covered during sleep.

- His feet should be touching the bottom of the cot (to prevent him sliding down beneath the covers) with the covers no higher than his shoulders.

- The covers should be tucked under the mattress so that they cannot move over your baby's face.

- Excess toys, quilts, or comforters should be removed from the cot.

- Ensure that your baby's environment is smoke-free.

- Avoid your baby becoming overheated from too much clothing, the room temperature being too high, or the cot being close to a heat source.

- Do not sleep with your baby on a sofa or armchair.

- Do not share the bed with your baby if you have drunk alcohol or have taken medicines or drugs that can make you less aware, and if you smoke, are obese, or are particularly tired.

5

Sleepless toddlers and preschool children (1–4 years)

➲ Key points

◆ Many children of this age are difficult to get to sleep at bedtime and/ or wake in the night insisting on their parents presence.

◆ These problems can be prevented or, if already established, treated in various ways.

✖ Myth versus fact

Myth: Bedtime and night-time waking problems are an inevitable phase in young children that parents have to endure until they—hopefully—stop.

Facts: Often such problems can be prevented or treated by means of appropriate measures on the part of the parents.

Settling and night waking problems are the main sleep problems in children (other than babies) under the age of about 4. Sometimes such problems persist until later than this. The main signs are rapid settling and return to sleep when the comforting conditions that your child has come to associate with going to sleep are provided. These **sleep onset associations** may be objects such as the cot, favourite toys, or other 'comfort' or 'transitional' objects, but frequently they involve the parent's presence, i.e. being held, rocked, or nursed. At least in most families in western society, a problem arises if the child cannot go to sleep at bedtime, and/or if he cannot get back to sleep after waking during the night without associations that involve the parents' presence and comforting attention (see Chapter 4).

A **consistent evening routine**, with a wind-down period of activities as bed-time approaches (as also described in Chapter 4), is very important at this age and indeed beyond. Difficulties at bedtime may also be related to inappropriate **patterns of daytime napping** (see Chapter 1), i.e. too little or too much day-time napping for the child's age or, alternatively, a nap too near to bedtime.

Bedtime struggles and other settling difficulties often continue after the age of 3 or thereabouts, especially when a child moves from a cot to a bed and can move around more easily. Many parents are familiar with bedtime delaying tactics in which their child asks for drinks or more stories, expresses fear at the prospect of bed, or steadfastly refuses to go to bed. Commonly, this problem is maintained or made worse if parents are unable or unwilling to establish and consistently enforce rules for going to bed and settling to sleep, i.e. to **set limits**. A clue to the nature of the problem can be the child's willing-ness to settle with one parent rather than the other, or with the babysitter or with someone else who can set limits. The problem is likely to be made worse if parents lose their temper, or threaten or punish the child, who then comes to associate bedtime with upset and fear. The risk of this happening is increased if parents are emotionally upset for whatever reason, such as marital discord.

Setting limits is only appropriate if the child is physiologically capable of going to sleep at the required time. Both children and adults have a period later in the day when their tendency to sleep is at its lowest (the 'forbidden zone'). This is followed by a period of least alertness leading to sleep onset. Understandably, if the child is put to bed while still wide awake, he will resist (perhaps vigorously). Events leading up to bedtime should be arranged so that the child goes to bed when he is 'sleepy tired'.

Observing these sorts of principles may prevent significant settling and trou-blesome night-time waking problems in toddlers and preschool children, but if this has not been the case, and especially if such problems are well estab-lished to the distress of parents and perhaps other family members, certain behavioural (i.e. non-medication) methods can be employed, which have been shown to be very effective in many cases.

Some of these treatments are more acceptable to some families than others, depending on how strict they feel able to be in putting them into practice. In all cases, it is important that the treatment programme is implemented with conviction and is seen through, despite possible setbacks, especially in its early stages when things can get worse before they get better. In such circumstances, parents may well need support and encouragement from the advising therapist to persist. Sometimes parents may feel that they have already undertaken this type of treatment and that it has failed. However, detailed enquiry may well reveal that actually the wrong choice of treatment was made or that it was not carried out properly. This might have been the case because, for example, the child's mother was emotionally incapable of what was required or was motivated to maintain the situation to preserve her child's dependence on her such that her own emotional needs were preserved. At one extreme, a child's presence in the parents' bed may be welcomed by one of them because it limits intimate contact with the other.

Some **ways of promoting self-soothing** (i.e. teaching the child to go to sleep at bedtime, and to go back to sleep when he wakes in the night, without needing his parents with him) are described briefly as follows:

- After a short bedtime routine, put you child in his cot or bed, say good night, and leave the room. Do not go back unless you fear that he is ill or in danger. If he wakes and cries out for you in the night, go back briefly to check all is well, but do not interact in any way and then leave the room and do not return while he is crying, to avoid reinforcing his demands for your attention. Follow the same procedure if there are further episodes of crying.

- Although this method can be effective after only a matter of a few days, you may well feel too upset to use it, or other members of the family may be upset by the noise, which can intensify before matters improve. In this case, there are less determined ways of ignoring the crying by gradually reducing contact with your child when he cries out in the night. This can involve gradually reducing the distance between you and your child when you go in to see him, lessening the time each night that you spend with him when he cries out, or, when he cries out, checking him about every 10 minutes to reassure him briefly but without doing anything more than that.

- If your child is old enough to understand, rewarding him (e.g. by means of a star chart) can be an effective additional measure.

It may be necessary to try different methods to find the one that suits you and your child best. However, the possible value of each method should be explored fully by implementing it with conviction and not abandoning it half way through. This may require the support of your health visitor or another professional adviser.

📄 Case study

Settling problems

For the previous year, the parents of a 3-year-od girl had been upset by her refusal to go to sleep at bedtime. The problem was getting worse to the extent that she was still awake in the early hours of the morning. Then she became reluctant to get up for nursery school and was tetchy during the day.

The parents were constantly tired and irritable. Different advice from other family members and friends was unhelpful and they eventually consulted their doctor who enlisted the help of a local child psychologist with a special interest in sleep disorders. She concluded that there were various ways in which the parents' handling of the problem could be improved.

The girl had been in the habit of watching exciting videos downstairs until quite late in the evening, after which she had to be put to bed rather forcefully. This was usually done by her mother who joined her in her bed, often issuing threats in an attempt to make her settle. When father took his turn, he adopted a less stern but equally ineffective approach.

Overall, the psychologist felt that the girl was overstimulated before bed-time and also that her problem behaviour was being given far too much attention, being reinforced in the process rather than being discouraged. In addition, the parents' efforts were considered inconsistent from night to night and between the two of them.

With support and encouragement, the parents were able to correct these shortcomings, including encouraging their daughter to fall asleep without them being with her and, with 4 weeks of persistent effort on their part, the bedtime problem was gradually solved.

📄 Case study

Troublesome night-time waking

The parents of a 4-year-old girl with a severe learning disability said that from birth she had tended to wake up every hour or so for long periods. More recently, she would wander about the house in the middle of the night and sometimes injured herself doing so. Sleeping medicine had not worked and seemed instead to make her sleepy during the day. Initially, they assumed that this sleep problem was an inevitable part of her basic condition and that any further attempts at treatment would not work so, for want of a better idea, they had resorted to taking her into their own bed where she usually slept until morning.

However, they became so dissatisfied with this arrangement that they asked the advice of their doctor again, who was able to refer them to a sleep disorders clinic for children. The first recommendation was that they should return their child to her own bed whenever she came into their room or wandered elsewhere at night. They were warned that they would need to be insistent about this, not to interact with her in doing so, and to expect an initial worsening of the problem. Telephone support from a member of the clinic staff was arranged for use whenever necessary.

On the first night, the child was taken back to her bed and told to sleep there, which she did quickly without being upset. She came out of her room again several times later that night, but each time was settled back in her own bed, resisting only slightly. This procedure was followed for a further week, during which time she gradually came out of her room less often until she stopped doing so completely. Occasionally, she would call out if she woke up, but her parents simply called back reassuringly and this seemed to be sufficient for her to be able to go back to sleep. After a further fortnight or so she stopped calling out altogether.

Her parents were delighted with this result, which, although they knew that such treatment often worked in other children, they had not expected on the assumption that it wouldn't be helpful in children with a learning disability, especially when the sleep problem had lasted such a long time.

6

School-aged children who can't sleep

➲ Key points

◆ The possible causes of sleeplessness at this age tend to be different from those in younger children, although there may be overlap to some extent.

◆ Emotional factors may play a prominent role, but other possibilities of a more physical nature should also be considered.

✖ Myth versus fact

Myth: Nightmares may well indicate a serious underlying emotional problem.

Fact: This is not usually the case if the nightmares are infrequent, but psychological help is needed if there is a strong suggestion that your child cannot sleep because he is persistently distressed in this or other ways.

Difficulty getting to sleep

Some of the causes of sleeplessness in pre-school children may still apply in older children, but other factors become more relevant with increasing age.

Night-time fears

Night-time fears are common from very early childhood onwards, although, in keeping with cognitive development, the content of the fears changes from aspects of the immediate environment (e.g. shadows or noises) to imaginary objects (ghosts or monsters) or the dark, to more realistic and specific fears concerning the child's own health. Such fears do not usually persist and require only reassurance and comfort until they cease.

In some children, the fears are very intense and persistent, and therefore need special attention. The cause of the fear should be investigated. A night-time fear may be one aspect of an anxiety state, including post-traumatic stress disorder, in which case the child may also suffer from nightmares. The content of the fear or nightmare can be revealing, suggesting the reason for the child's emotional upset. Other sleep disturbances (e.g. alarming hypnagogic hallucinations; see Chapter 13) may be the cause of the night-time fears. Obviously, it is important to differentiate between a child who is reluctant to go to bed because he is genuinely afraid and one who is pretending to be afraid as a delaying tactic.

Behavioural treatment can be very effective for severe night-time fears. The child should be helped to feel positive about going to bed, and should not go to bed so early that he lies awake in a fearful state.

Worries and anxiety

Worries and anxiety about daytime matters such as school or problems at home may cause difficulties in getting to sleep or staying asleep. The original source of concern may no longer exist but the difficulty in falling asleep may persist because the child has developed the habit of lying awake in bed in an agitated state ('conditioned insomnia').

Sympathetic discussion of a child's worries, attention to the source of concern if possible, and ways of helping him to relax at night may well help. More specific psychiatric measures will be needed if the child has an anxiety or depressive disorder, or if there is evidence of serious problems within the family.

Restless legs syndrome

Restless legs syndrome (see Chapter 12) consists of disagreeable leg sensations with an irresistible urge to move the legs, causing difficulty getting to sleep in people of all ages. It is often accompanied by periodic limb movements (see Chapter 14). 'Growing pains', said to be a cause of sleep difficulties in otherwise healthy children, is an ill-defined condition. When they occur around bedtime, restless legs syndrome is a possibility.

Other causes

Other possible causes of difficulty in getting to sleep (according to parents) at the required time are an 'owl' sleep–wake pattern (see Chapter 1) or an unusual constitutional tendency to insomnia dating from an early age ('idiopathic or child-onset insomnia'). 'Conditioned insomnia' can also occur at almost any age, where the original cause of not being able to sleep has ceased to exist but the habit of not sleeping well has persisted.

Night waking

Certain parasomnias (see later chapters) often develop at this age but they will be a cause of insomnia only if (unusually) they occur frequently each night.

Early morning waking

Again, at this age, and perhaps later, there are a number of possible reasons for waking up well before most other people and not being able to get back to sleep again. These include being disturbed by noises within the house or outside, not needing as much sleep as other people ('short sleeper'), a 'lark'-type of sleep–wake pattern, or habitually having gone to sleep unusually early so that sleep requirements have been met by the early hours ('advanced sleep-phase syndrome').

📄 Case study

Night-time fears

A little boy, age 5, had always slept well. He readily settled to sleep each night in his own room and slept soundly until it was time to get up. However, starting just a few weeks before, he had began to refuse to go to bed by himself and became very distressed when his mother or father left him in his room. Often, he followed them downstairs crying and strongly resisted being taken back. During the night, after having eventually fallen asleep, he woke up again in an agitated state and insisted on joining his parents in their bed. Even during the day, he seemed afraid to go upstairs. Understandably, these changes in his behaviour were upsetting to his parents who had begun to worry that there might be something seriously wrong with him psychologically.

He was referred by the family doctor to a child psychologist with experience of treating sleep problems. She managed to find out that he had become afraid that there might be something harmful in his bedroom although he couldn't say what and it wasn't clear why he had started to feel this way. Increasingly, he had come to misinterpret shadows and noises elsewhere in the house as evidence of some frightening presence. In other respects he was well. There were no problems in the family or at school to explain the change in him.

The psychologist advised the boy's parents to reassure him at bedtime that he was safe, that there was nothing to harm him, and that they were always nearby. Telling him that lots of children are anxious in this way for a time was thought to be likely to make him feel less strange. They were advised to discuss his fears with him (preferably during the day rather than just at bedtime when the matter might prey on his mind) and to plan with him ways of coping with his fears by imagining something pleasant to help him relax if he started to feel panicky.

He was also to be encouraged not to cry out and to stay in his bedroom if he was afraid during the night. This was to avoid him becoming conditioned to his parents being in his room. He was to be rewarded for 'being brave' if he controlled his fears in this way. Other measures consisted of having a comfort object with him in bed and (at least to begin with) allowing him a nightlight and leaving his bedroom door partly open. Avoiding watching frightening TV programmes before bedtime was not an issue as he had never done this.

Both the child and his parents were able to follow this advice, although initially they needed some support from the psychologist to persist when, to begin with, he became more anxious. However, within a month he was able to get to sleep readily and to sleep soundly again.

7

Sleeplessness (insomnia) in adolescents

 Key points

- Similar to the situation in children at a younger age, worries may be a cause of sleeping difficulties in teenagers, but body-clock changes combined with lifestyle choices may also be a cause.

- Alterations in sleep patterns for these reasons should not be mistaken for difficult behaviour. If serious, they call for treatment not recriminations.

- There may be other, quite different, causes at this age, requiring special advice or treatment.

✗ Myth versus fact

Myth: Many teenagers do not go to sleep until late and are difficult to get up in the morning, as well as lying in bed at weekends until very late, because of bad habits.

Fact: This is not necessarily the case. This pattern may be an actual sleep disorder that is partly due to physiological changes at puberty and which requires treatment.

In general, older children sleep very efficiently before the onset of puberty and can be very alert during the day. Adolescents are often different in these respects and high rates of insomnia have been described consistently at this stage of development.

A particularly important cause of difficulty in getting to sleep and resultant sleepiness during the day (see Chapter 9, including the case illustration) is a change in the body clock at puberty, which shifts the time that you are ready for sleep until later than it used to be. A combination of this change and the habit of staying up late anyway for social activities (or perhaps to study into the early hours) can easily result in not being able to get to sleep until late at night (so-called **delayed sleep-phase syndrome** or DSPS (see Chapter 9).

The difficulty in falling asleep can be severe, lasting until the early hours. Concern about not getting enough sleep is likely to make the problem worse. As not enough sleep has been obtained by the time it is necessary to get up for school, college, or work, attempts to wake the teenager may be met with resistance.

It is all too easy for parents to interpret the going to sleep late and wanting to stay in bed in the morning (as well as sleeping in late at weekends in what is actually a vain attempt to make up for the loss of sleep during the week) as 'typical difficult adolescent behaviour'. In fact, DSPS and its effects on behaviour have a physiological basis that needs to be corrected in various ways by re-timing the sleep phase rather than simply remonstrating with the young person.

The most appropriate management of DSPS is usually to advance the sleep phase gradually, first by bringing the time of waking forward and then the bedtime, including weekends. There are good prospects for improvement provided the treatment programme is followed carefully. If highly irregular sleep–wake patterns are just one aspect of a lack of routine in family life, or if the young person is not motivated to change, the outcome will be less than satisfactory unless basic attitudes can be changed.

It is, of course, important to distinguish DSPS from other reasons why a teenager may not want to get up and go to school, such as the more usual form of refusal to go to school, depression, chronic fatigue syndrome, or substance abuse.

American surveys have shown that only about 20% of adolescents get the recommended 9 hours of sleep on school nights and almost half sleep less than 8 hours. At least once a week, a quarter of those studied fell asleep in school and those who got insufficient sleep were more likely to get lower grades. The other possible harmful effects of insufficient sleep were described in Chapter 2. Parents, teachers, and teenagers themselves need to be able to recognize the signs of poor sleep and, collectively, do something to solve the problem. Otherwise, both immediate and long-term educational and social consequences can be serious.

Difficulties in getting off to sleep and broken sleep can be the result of worries about daytime demands, relationship problems, or other causes of stress, all of which are thought to be common in adolescence. Alcohol, nicotine, and caffeine-containing drinks, especially coffee, of which surprisingly large amount may be consumed, can cause difficulties in getting off to sleep or broken sleep later in the night. The other psychiatric and medical conditions mentioned earlier may need to be considered, as well as medication effects. Possible drug misuse is particularly relevant at this age and is capable of producing a range of sleep problems including insomnia.

8

Excessive daytime sleepiness

➔ Key points

◆ Being so sleepy during the day that your child cannot function properly is not uncommon.

◆ Excessive sleepiness may be misinterpreted as a different type of problem such as laziness.

◆ There are many possible causes that should be considered: not getting enough sleep, poor quality sleep for various reasons, or having one of a number of a conditions that make you sleep much more than normal.

◆ As in the case of other sleep problems, it is important that the cause in your child is discovered so that the right advice and, if necessary, treatment can be given.

✖ Myth versus fact

Myth: Being so sleepy that it interferes with your everyday activities is rare.

Fact: Many people (including children—and especially adolescents) are seriously affected by being excessively sleepy during the day.

The following are some questions you should ask yourself about your child's sleep–wake pattern and related matters to help decide the nature and cause of his excessive sleepiness.

1. What is the nature and degree of his sleepiness?

    ◆ In what ways exactly is your child too sleepy?

    ◆ How long does he usually sleep at night? How does this compare with the average for a child of his age (see Chapter 1)?

    ◆ Does he sleep soundly or is his sleep interrupted a lot at night?

    ◆ Is it extremely difficult to wake him in the morning in spite of his having gone to sleep at a reasonable time?

    ◆ Does he have to take naps during the day?

2. Is it delayed sleep phase syndrome?

    ◆ Is he unable to get to sleep until very late at night?

    ◆ Does he have particular difficulty waking up in the morning?

    ◆ Compared with weekdays, does he sleep in very late at weekends, for example until well into the afternoon?

3. Does he have obstructive sleep apnoea?

    ◆ Does he snore a lot or breathe noisily in other ways at night?

    ◆ Does he seem to stop breathing repeatedly at night?

    ◆ Does he appear to have large tonsils and adenoids?

4. Does he have restless legs syndrome or periodic leg movements in his sleep?

    ◆ Has your child complained of uncomfortable feelings in his legs in the evenings?

    ◆ Do his legs kick repeatedly during sleep?

5. Does he suffer from narcolepsy?

    ◆ Is he unable to stop falling asleep repeatedly during the day?

    ◆ Does he ever collapse or feel weak in any way when amused, excited, or alarmed?

◆ Has he ever described strange experiences when drifting off to sleep or when waking up, including briefly not being able to move?

6. Is it seasonal affective disorder or some other type of intermittent sleepiness?

◆ Is your child very sleepy and different from his usual self during the winter months?

◆ At any time of the year, does he have periods of being extremely sleepy (perhaps for many days at a time) but being his usual self in between?

◆ Is your daughter very sleepy around the time of her monthly periods?

7. What has his general health and behaviour been like?

◆ Does your child have any illness or disorder that disturbs his sleep a lot at night?

◆ Does he take any medication that seems to make him sleepy during the day?

◆ Does he at present have any other sort of illness or disorder?

◆ Is he thought to have attention-deficit hyperactivity disorder (ADHD)?

◆ Has he had any serious illness in the past after which his sleep pattern changed?

Excessive daytime sleepiness (EDS) has been a neglected sleep problem

In the Introduction to this book, mention was made of some people who in the past had drawn attention to the importance of children's sleep disorders well before modern interest in the subject had begun to develop.

In 1545, Thomas Phaire drew attention to what would now be called sleeplessness, nightmares, infantile colic and bedwetting, all of which are fairly obvious problems. In 1892, William Osler described noisy breathing as a prominent feature of obstructive sleep apnoea. Clement Dukes, in 1905, was mainly concerned about various serious effects of the lack of sleep. However, overall, relatively little attention was paid to excessive sleepiness and its effects, although Osler was mindful of the dulling effects on daytime behaviour of obstructive sleep apnoea caused by its disruptive effects on sleep.

It was Anders and his colleagues in 1978 at Stanford University who laid particular emphasis on the problem of excessive sleepiness. They chided doctors for not paying it more attention, saying that '*the "sleepy child" has been ignored by physicians, attracting medical attention only after daytime sleepiness has seriously impaired education*'.

EDS can easily be misinterpreted

Matters have improved since that time; for example, there is now a growing awareness that many teenagers suffer from being very sleepy. However, there is still the risk that, compared with more compelling types of sleep disturbance, this particular sleep problem will not come to medical attention or that sleepiness will be misinterpreted as laziness, disinterest, misbehaviour, chronic fatigue syndrome, or some other condition, even limited intellectual ability, especially if it has persisted for some time.

This risk is made more likely by the fact that, whereas sleepy adults are usually slowed down by their condition, sleepy children's activity levels may increase accompanied by poor concentration or impulsive behaviour, sometimes to the extent that they are mistakenly diagnosed as having ADHD, without the realization that the cause of their problem behaviour is a sleep disorder.

Various types of sleep problem or disorder (described elsewhere in this book) have been described as acting in this way: insufficient sleep, obstructive sleep apnoea, periodic limb movements in sleep, and narcolepsy. Treatment of such children should aim mainly to correct their sleep disorder rather than target their daytime behaviour with 'stimulant' drugs of the type often used for ADHD.

The signs are that many very sleepy children, even those in whom the cause is definitely physical (such as obstructive sleep apnoea or narcolepsy) are not assessed medically or are only eventually assessed after a long delay because the problem has been misconstrued.

How common is EDS?

Excessive sleepiness seems to be a problem mainly in older children and especially in adolescents. However, because of the problems of recognition mentioned above, just how common it is at these ages is not known.

It cannot be rare in view of its many underlying causes, some of which are individually far from rare. The figure of 5% sometimes quoted for the number of young people with EDS is likely to be wide of the mark if only because of the high proportion of teenagers found in the surveys mentioned in Chapter 7 who often fall asleep at school. Indeed, when asked, many teenagers complain about excessive sleepiness, but it has been claimed that very many more than those who seek help are likely to be suffering in this way, mainly as a result of long-term lack of sleep or 'sleep debt'. The adverse effects of this can be wide-ranging, from underperformance at school, college, or work to road traffic accidents and other mishaps, as well as antisocial behaviour. Sometimes, such problems are made worse by the use of stimulants to stay awake, or by alcohol or sedative drugs to get to sleep.

Is it really EDS?

It is important to establish that the problem really is excessive sleepiness. 'Tiredness' can mean a number of things. Ideally, sleepiness (i.e. needing to sleep) should be distinguished from fatigue or lethargy (which do not necessarily indicate a need to sleep) for which different explanations are likely including physical illnesses (such as anaemia), other signs of which can usually be seen. Young people with chronic fatigue syndrome may have sleep problems,

Table 8.1 Causes of EDS in children and adolescents

Reason for sleepiness	Cause
Insufficient sleep	Sleeplessness or insomnia
	Erratic sleep–wake patterns
	Delayed sleep phase syndrome
Disturbed night-time sleep	Substances that interfere with sound sleep (e.g. caffeine, alcohol, nicotine)
	Obstructive sleep apnoea
	Illicit drugs (including withdrawal symptoms)
	Medical and psychiatric disorders
	Other sleep disorders (frequent parasomnias, periodic limb movements in sleep)
Increased need for sleep	Narcolepsy
	Idiopathic central nervous system hypersomnia
	Depression
	Substance abuse
	Kleine–Levin syndrome (intermittent sleepiness)
	Menstruation-related hypersomnia (intermittent sleepiness)

but these rarely take the form of true EDS. Occasionally, someone will spend long periods in bed, seeming to be asleep much of the time (but not actually sleeping) in order to escape from an emotionally difficult situation.

The various causes of EDS can be grouped as follows (see Table 8.1):

♦ insufficient or lack of sleep;

♦ disrupted (poor-quality) sleep;

♦ conditions in which there is an increased need for sleep.

Further details of each of these causes are given in Chapters 9–11.

9

Lack of sleep as a cause of being very sleepy

→ Key points

◆ If your child is often very sleepy, the first thing to determine is whether he is getting enough sleep for his age.

◆ Try to assess how many hours he is actually asleep at night, not just how long he spends in bed.

◆ Consider the possible reasons for actual loss of sleep (discussed in Chapters 5–7), depending on your child's age.

✖ Myth versus fact

Myth: You can get used to having less sleep than previously.

Fact: This is very unlikely. Most people (including children) will be affected by not having enough sleep. They may forget how they used to feel and be pleasantly surprised how much better they are if their sleep improves.

Lack of sleep is the main cause of being sleepy during the day. There are many ways in which this situation can arise.

The many causes discussed in the preceding chapters of sleeplessness or insomnia, sufficient to significantly reduce sleep below what is needed to function properly during the day, have to be considered as a possible explanation of why a child is excessively sleepy.

The possibilities include a disturbance of your child's circadian sleep–wake cycle. This may take the form of irregular sleep–wake schedules or, more usually, delayed sleep-phase syndrome (DSPS) (see Chapter 7), which deserves further mention here because it is common, especially in adolescents, and is potentially very harmful. Both of these circadian sleep–wake disorders cause a child's sleep to be inadequate.

At any age, the time at which your child falls asleep may become delayed during a period of illness. From an early age, a more persistent delay may develop because of repeated disputes at bedtime about going to bed.

In adolescence, the problem arises from the combination of the body clock change at puberty, which tends to make it more difficult to go to sleep than at an earlier age (see Chapter 1) and a tendency to stay up late for entertainment or social reasons or for study. After a time (the length of which varies with the individual), the sleep phase becomes physiologically delayed with the result that it becomes impossible to go to sleep earlier by choice, in spite of feeling tired and having been awake for a long time.

By the time it is necessary to get up for school, college, or work, your child's sleep needs (at least 9 hours a night) have not been met. The result is considerable difficulty getting up in the morning, tiredness, or actually falling asleep during the day, and quite possibly irritability or other unwelcome behaviour.

In these circumstances, entreaties to go to bed at a sensible time and get up at the required time are likely to be ineffective. Correction of the problem requires a change of lifestyle and other measures mentioned below; however, these may be difficult to achieve without strong motivation and, if necessary, firm parental control of the situation.

The features of DSPS to look for are persistently severe difficulty in getting to sleep, uninterrupted sound sleep, great difficulty getting up for school or work, and sleepiness and underfunctioning, especially during the first part of the day, giving way to alertness in the evening and early hours. The abnormal sleep pattern is maintained by sleeping in very late when able to do so at weekends and during holidays.

Treatment consists of gradually and consistently changing the sleep phase to an appropriate time. This can be achieved by slowly advancing the sleep phase (e.g. by 15 min a day) where the phase delay is about 3 hours or less. In more severe forms of DSPS, it is necessary to delay the sleep phase progressively in 3-hour steps 'around the clock'.

Early morning exposure to daylight and a firm agreement with your child to maintain the new pattern of social activities and sleep will help to maintain the new sleep pattern. Melatonin, taken in the evening, may also be helpful in getting your child to get to sleep at a more appropriate time.

Achieving and maintaining an improved sleep–wake pattern by these means may not be easy. The difficulties are increased if a child has a vested interest in maintaining his abnormal sleep pattern, for example to avoid attending school.

Case study

Delayed sleep-phase syndrome

The mother of a 15-year-old girl had been taken to court by her local education authority and convicted because her daughter had failed to attend school consistently over the previous 12 months. The mother appealed against this conviction on the grounds that her daughter had something wrong with her sleep that made it particularly difficult for her to get up in the morning but this was treated with some scepticism.

The help of a sleep expert was obtained and enquiries revealed that for the last 3 years the girl had been going to bed progressively later and later as a result of reading, watching TV and doing homework in her bedroom until late at night, during which time she usually drank at least two mugs of coffee. Eventually, although she went to bed at about 10 p.m., she was unable to get to sleep until 2–3 a.m., after which she slept soundly until her mother's attempts to wake her, which she strongly resisted. Increasingly, she would go back to sleep and either not go to school or arrive late.

When at school, she was described as 'looking awful' and being 'very morose' and sometimes she fell asleep in class. The standard of her work was much lower than it had been previously when she was keen to succeed academically. At weekends and during holidays, she had the same difficulty getting to sleep and was in the habit of sleeping in until about midday or later.

These features of her sleep pattern were typical of the recognized sleep disorder called delayed sleep phase syndrome, which is common in adolescence and is the result of a combination of body clock changes at puberty (which makes it difficult to get to sleep than at an earlier age) and habitually staying up late. Having to get up in time for school meant that she had become severely short of sleep ('sleep debt'). The problem, therefore, was physiological and was not 'difficult adolescent behaviour' or an attempt to avoid school.

When this had been explained to the court, her mother's conviction was quashed, and the girl was started on treatment aimed at retiming her sleep phase. She also stopped drinking coffee late in the day, which would have been adding to her insomnia problem. Soon, she was able to get to sleep at midnight at the latest and had much less difficulty getting up in the morning. From then on, her progress at school was good.

10

Excessive sleepiness due to disturbed sleep

→ Key points

◆ Sometimes overnight sleep is not refreshing, not because it is too short but because it is superficial and of poor quality.

◆ There are various causes of poor quality sleep, each of which calls for different advice and possibly treatment.

◆ Each cause should be able to be identified by means of careful enquiries and then treated successfully.

✖ Myth versus fact

Myth: If your child sleeps long enough for his age, he will be all right during the day.

Fact: The quality of his sleep is as important as how many hours he sleeps.

If your child is very sleepy during the day, despite seeming to sleep the usual length of time for his age, this suggests that his sleep is of poor quality and is not restoring him sufficiently.

Poor-quality sleep can result from frequent awakenings or less obvious arousals including brief interruptions (or 'fragmentation') of sleep. Sleep may be disturbed by a number of factors.

Various substances can disrupt sleep, some of which may be consumed in adolescence. The most common is caffeine, which is contained not only in coffee but also in cola drinks, some stimulant energy drinks, tea, and even chocolate. Coffee intake can be considerable while socializing in the evenings, sometimes with the intention of staying awake until late. This is likely to make it difficult eventually to get to sleep and to sleep soundly, partly because it may cause frequent trips to the toilet. Alcohol may make you sleepy but later in the night it is likely to disturb your sleep including making you dream more. Disrupted sleep can also be caused by nicotine and various illicit drugs, not only while they are being used but also during their withdrawal.

Sleep can be disrupted by many **medical and psychiatric disorders**, and sometimes by the **medications** prescribed for them. Obstructive sleep apnoea (OSA) is an example of a medical condition that can seriously disrupt sleep. It is worth saying more about this condition because it is quite common and can affect a child's learning and behaviour.

Obstructive sleep apnoea

At least 2% of children in general have some degree of OSA, mainly those between the age of 2 and 6 years. It occurs much more often than this in children with certain forms of learning disability, such as Down syndrome, or facial deformity. There are important differences between OSA in children and adults. The typical adult with OSA is an obese, middle-aged male who snores very loudly and underfunctions during the day, with general slowing down of his activities. In contrast, most children with OSA are not obese (although this is increasing as a factor as more and more children are becoming obese), and the usual cause is large tonsils and adenoids, removal of which can be beneficial. Also, the number of boys and girls with OSA is about equal, and children may have generally noisy breathing rather than the loud snoring heard in adults, and with less obvious interruptions in their breathing. Moreover, the result of sleep disruption may well be overactivity and other disruptive behaviour, rather than obvious sleepiness during the day.

The following factors that, in combination at night, suggest that a child has OSA are:

◆ very noisy breathing or actual snoring at night (although only about one in five children who snores most nights has this condition);

◆ other signs of breathing difficulties during sleep such as vigorous movements of the chest and abdomen caused by attempts to overcome the obstruction and get air into the chest;

◆ unusual sleeping positions including sleeping with the head tilted backwards to help get air past the obstruction;

◆ very restless sleep, profuse sweating, bedwetting, and sudden distressing awakenings related to difficulty breathing.

Daytime features include breathing through the mouth because of difficulty breathing through the nose, headaches, and being in a bad mood on wakening, as well as the behaviour problems already mentioned.

Physical examination may reveal the anatomical cause of the obstruction (usually enlarged tonsils and adenoids). Special imaging studies are required in more complicated cases and sleep studies (polysomnography) with various measures of breathing function are needed to assess the severity of the obstruction. OSA sometimes seems to provoke other sleep disorders such as nightmares and, in children genetically predisposed to them (see Chapter 15), arousal disorders. Treatment is essential to counteract or prevent physical and psychological complications. This usually consists of removal of the tonsils and adenoids.

Finally, sleep can be disrupted by other sleep disorders. Frequent parasomnias are likely to be obvious, but periodic limb movements in sleep (see Chapter 14)—now considered to be more important in childhood than previously thought—are much more subtle in their effects on sleep.

📄 Case study

Obstructive sleep apnoea

The mother of a 10-year-old boy went to see their GP because, although she said his sleep had been disturbed for as long as she could remember, his snoring, gasping and choking noises at night had now become so loud that she and her husband were constantly woken up by them, even though her son slept in his own room. When she went to his bedroom to try to stop him making so much noise, she had noticed that he repeatedly stopped breathing, sometimes for an alarming length of time. He also often slept with his head tipped back and was generally a very restless sleeper. Recently, he had wet the bed occasionally after previously being dry from about the age of 4. Both she and his teachers said that he was very sleepy during the day and generally irritable. His progress at school was somewhat below average.

The boy was referred to a paediatrician with a special interest in respiratory disorders who confirmed the GP's suspicion that the boy was suffering from a fairly severe degree of OSA caused by enlarged tonsils and adenoids, which could clearly be seen when his throat was examined. It was thought that this was a long-standing condition, but that it had worsened in recent times. His daytime sleepiness and irritability (and his occasional bedwetting) was thought likely to be due to the disturbance of his sleep, which was evident when overnight sleep studies were performed in hospital.

Following the removal of his tonsils and adenoids, the boy began to sleep normally, much to his parents' relief. He was no longer sleepy during the day, he became generally more amenable, his schoolwork improved, and he stopped wetting the bed again.

11

Sleep disorders that make you sleep too much

➔ Key points

♦ There are various conditions, each with recognizable characteristics, in which prolonged or otherwise excessive sleep is an intrinsic part of their nature, rather than a consequence of them.

♦ In some of these conditions, the sleepiness is continuous; in others, it comes and goes at intervals.

✖ Myth versus fact

Myth: Sleeping repeatedly or for long periods is probably just a bad habit or laziness.

Fact: This is often mistakenly thought of children with medical disorders in which the need to sleep is abnormal.

Myth: If a child goes through periods of being very sleepy and yet is normal in between, it is likely to be a psychological problem.

Fact: This is not necessarily the case and a medical condition should be suspected.

Narcolepsy

Narcolepsy is a neurological disorder caused by low levels of a chemical in the brain called hypocretin (or orexin), mainly affecting rapid eye movement (REM) sleep. It is not the rarity it was once supposed and is also not a psychological condition as was suggested at one time. It has been estimated to occur in perhaps 1 in 2000 of the population, and in about a third of these, it starts in childhood or adolescence, although unfortunately the diagnosis is often not made for several years. The reasons for this are that the symptoms may be subtle in their early stages, or may be misinterpreted as laziness or a psychological disorder, or they may be overshadowed by the child's emotional upset at having the condition.

📄 Case study

Narcolepsy

A 14-year-old girl had been perfectly well all her life, but then, for no apparent reason, began to feel very sleepy most of the time and kept falling asleep for brief periods, even when she was actively engaged in doing things at home or at school. Soon after, she also began to feel weak and to fall to the ground (without losing consciousness) when she was amused or suddenly startled. She then described that, when drifting off to sleep at night, she often had odd distortions of her vision and a feeling that she couldn't move for a matter of several seconds. Not surprisingly, she found these experiences very disturbing. In other respects she was fine. She had been a happy girl who was making very good progress at school. No one else in the family had any illnesses or disorders of any significance.

At the request of her GP, she was seen by a paediatric neurologist. On the basis of the story, backed up by overnight sleep studies, a multiple sleep latency test (see Chapter 2), and some blood tests, he diagnosed narcolepsy syndrome, which in her case was somewhat unusual in view of the fact that she had displayed all of the classical features of the condition in rapid succession.

Treatment was started with the combination of a stimulant drug to combat the sleepiness and, for the other parts of the syndrome, a drug normally used for depression. She soon made a good response, although some of her symptoms remained to some extent. Clearly, it was important (with her permission) to explain the nature of her condition to her family, teachers, and peers to avoid misunderstandings about her symptoms.

The early signs of narcolepsy are very variable and some time usually elapses before the classic features of the condition appear. These are:

◆ daytime sleep attacks of irresistible sleep;

◆ general sleepiness because night-time sleep is disrupted;

- attacks of cataplexy in which the child becomes weak (and often falls down), usually when emotionally aroused;

- strange sensations when going off to sleep (hypnagogic hallucinations) or when waking up (hypnopompic hallucinations);

- brief episodes of not being able to move when going to sleep or waking up (sleep paralysis).

The combination of these features is referred to as the 'narcolepsy syndrome'. Not all of these components of the syndrome necessarily develop. The key symptoms are sleep attacks and cataplexy; the rest occur—not uncommonly— by themselves in healthy people (see Chapter 13).

Narcolepsy should be suspected in any young person who is excessively sleepy during the day without an obvious explanation, but repeated assessment may be required at intervals before a definite diagnosis can be made, including its distinction from other forms of sleepiness.

Narcolepsy is a persistent and disturbing condition for which careful treatment with medication (stimulants, such as modafinil, for the sleepiness and other drugs for the other features) is prescribed. Other important measures include support and advice about education, career, and psycho-social matters.

Other causes of excessive sleepiness

Idiopathic hypersomnia is another (unusual) neurological cause of excessive sleepiness, but without the characteristic features of narcolepsy. It often starts in childhood or adolescence and can run in families. In this condition, waking up properly in the morning is particularly difficult, despite having had a sound night's sleep, perhaps for longer than most people. After waking, drowsiness and confusion can persist for some hours ('sleep drunkenness') and long unrefreshing naps may have to be taken during the day. Stimulant medication can be helpful.

Other causes of sustained sleepiness include **severe depression**. Most depressed people of any age suffer from insomnia, but many complain that they are excessively sleepy (as well as being fatigued). This excessive sleepiness may not simply be the result of not sleeping well. Successful antidepressant treatment usually improves the abnormal sleep pattern.

Various states of **drug intoxication**, as well as withdrawal from stimulant drugs, are other causes of excessive sleepiness. The same is true of **seasonal**

affective disorder (SAD), which occurs in the winter months in both children and adults. Accompanying problems include other types of sleeping difficulties, depression, fatigue, and overeating. Treatment includes exposure to bright light using a 'light box'.

A different pattern of intermittent excessive sleepiness is seen in **Kleine–Levin syndrome**. This relatively rare condition usually begins in the teenage years. Very long periods of excessive sleepiness (lasting many days or longer) alternate with periods of normality. Classically, during the sleepy periods, in the few hours that he is awake each day, the child behaves in an uncharacteristic and perhaps bizarre fashion by, for example, overeating and being disinhibited in other ways. Understandably, this condition may well be mistaken for a psychological disorder. Medication has little part to play but, fortunately, improvement tends to occur with age. In the meantime, it is obviously important to explain to all concerned that this is an illness and not a psychological disorder.

Disturbed sleep in girls, including intermittent excessive sleepiness, can be related to the **menstrual cycle** (possibly from an early age) in various ways such as an accompaniment of pre-menstrual tension or depression, or in the first few days of a period.

📄 Case study

Kleine–Levin syndrome

Over a period of about 18 months, a 10-year-old boy began to have recurrent periods (sometimes lasting weeks) of sleeping up to 14 hours a day. When awake, he began to behave in various bizarre and out-of-character ways including chasing his friend with a carving knife, stealing from the greengrocer, and using foul language. In between these periods, he became his usual normal self again.

Perhaps not surprisingly, his doctors initially thought that he had a psychiatric disorder, but his mother disputed this and thought it must somehow be a medical condition.

Sleep recordings showed that the long sleep periods were real and not pretend. This and the episodes of strange, unaccountable behaviour were considered typical of the Kleine–Levin syndrome, which is an obscure neurological disorder and not a psychiatric condition.

In this boy's case, treatment with lithium prevented further episodes.

12

Strange behaviour or experiences at night (parasomnias)

➔ Key points

♦ There are many different conditions in which children may behave strangely or have unusual experiences in relation to sleep.

♦ Although some may be dramatic and worrying to parents, they do not usually mean that the child is psychologically disturbed or medically ill in any way.

♦ Very often, parasomnias stop of their own accord after a while, but safety measures may be necessary in the meantime in some of them.

♦ Occasionally, sleep disorders of this type are part of a medical or psychological disorder that needs treatment in its own right.

♦ Many parasomnias can be grouped according to when at night they occur.

✖ Myth versus fact

Myth: Sleep is a highly quiescent state with very little happening.

Fact: This is not so. There are many possible ways in which behaviour and experience can be disturbed (sometimes dramatically) in relation to sleep, some of them quite common.

> **Myth:** Very strange behaviour or bizarre experiences at night must mean that a child has something seriously wrong with him.
>
> **Fact:** However dramatic the event, this is very rarely the case.
>
> **Myth:** You cannot do complicated things while you are still asleep.
>
> **Fact:** This is definitely not the case. For example, sleepwalkers sometimes do very complex things while still soundly asleep.

What are parasomnias?

Parasomnias can be thought of as unusual behaviour or strange experiences that occur predominantly or exclusively as you are going to sleep, during sleep, or when waking up.

Types of parasomnia

It is useful to divide the many childhood parasomnias into two broad categories:

◆ **Primary parasomnias** are sleep disorders in their own right. They can be classified according to the phase of sleep with which they are usually associated and therefore with the time at which they occur (see Table 12.1).

◆ **Secondary parasomnias** are manifestations of medical, behavioural, or psychiatric conditions (see Table 12.2).

Some basic points about parasomnias

In Chapter 1, Thomas Phaire's very limited but intriguing account of childhood parasomnias (and their curious recommended treatment) was mentioned. Much more is now known about this category of sleep disorders. In fact, 30 or so types are now officially recognized.

Parasomnias occur at all ages, but collectively they are more common in children than in adults. Frequently, they cause parents much concern and appear to be often confused with each other, with the result that inappropriate advice and treatment may be given.

Table 12.1 The main primary parasomnias and sleep phase in which they occur

Sleep phase	Parasomnia
When going to sleep initially (and sometimes after waking in the night)	Sleep starts Hypnagogic hallucinations Sleep paralysis Rhythmic movement disorder Restless legs syndrome
Early in the night (or later) in light non-rapid eye movement (NREM) sleep	Bruxism (teeth grinding) Periodic limb movements in sleep
Early in the night in deep NREM sleep: arousal disorders	Confusional arousals Sleepwalking Sleep terrors
Later in the night in rapid eye movement (REM) sleep	Nightmares REM sleep behaviour disorder (sometimes a secondary parasomnia)
When waking up	Hypnopompic hallucinations Sleep paralysis
Various times of the night	Sleeptalking Nocturnal enuresis

Table 12.2 Main secondary parasomnias

Origin	Parasomnia
Medical	Nocturnal epilepsies Other
Psychiatric or behavioural	Post-traumatic stress disorder parasomnias Nocturnal panic attacks Sleep-related eating disorders Dissociative states Malingering

Table 12.3 Comparison of the main usual features of arousal disorders, nightmares, and night-time seizures

Condition	Characteristics
Arousal disorders (confusional arousals, sleepwalking, and sleep terrors)	Common
	A family history is common
	Occur in first third of night (from deep NREM sleep)
	Often dramatic, with risk of injury
	Asleep at the time and often no waking
	Inaccessible and cannot be comforted
	No memory of events
	Confused if woken
	Variable frequency and duration
	Mostly cease spontaneously in time
Nightmares	Common
	No family history
	Occur late in night (in REM sleep)
	Injury unlikely
	Distressed and fully woken up by frightening and vividly recalled dream
	Accessible and needs comforting when awakes
	May take a while to calm down
	Usually infrequent and temporary
Epileptic seizures at night (there are various types only the more dramatic of which are likely to be confused with other parasomnias; the following are generalizations and there are many exceptions)	Much less common
	Variable family history
	Occur at variable times of night
	Injury unlikely
	Range of behaviour (often the same each time), possibly including strange movements and noises
	May or may not be confused during or after seizure, with or without memory of events
	Recovery can be prompt or prolonged
	Variable frequency and duration
	Outlook variable depending on type of epilepsy and underlying cause

In particular, arousal disorders such as sleepwalking or sleep terrors (see Chapter 15), nightmares (see Chapter 16) and some types of night-time epileptic seizures (see Chapter 18) can be mistaken for one another. Table 12.3 indicates the main ways in which these conditions differ.

The following general points about childhood parasomnias are worth making.

- A precise diagnosis is important as different parasomnias may well need contrasting types of treatment. Accurate diagnosis depends principally on a detailed account of the subjective and objective sequence of events from the start of the episode until it ends, as well as the circumstances in which the episode occurred, including its timing. Audio-visual recording (including the use by parents of home video systems) can be very helpful.

- The more dramatic forms of parasomnia understandably cause parents most concern but often unnecessarily, as most are benign in the sense that they are not a sign of a medical or psychological disorder.

- Especially when the range and features of sleep disorders is not sufficiently well known, parasomnias (and, for that matter, other sleep disorders) may well be misinterpreted as something other than what they really are (see Chapter 21).

- A child may have more than one kind of parasomnia or, indeed, more than type of one sleep disorder (e.g. obstructive sleep apnoea can be associated with sleepwalking).

- As many childhood primary parasomnias stop of their own accord within a few years if not before, children and parents can often be reassured about the future, although protective measures (e.g. in cases of severe headbanging or sleepwalking) may be required in the meantime.

- Specific treatment, including medication, is needed in only a minority of cases of primary parasomnia, but is likely to be needed for the underlying disorder in many of the secondary parasomnias.

- Research information on this point is limited, but a primary parasomnia may suggest a psychological problem if it is very frequent, unusually late when it first appears, persists beyond the age at which it usually stops, or follows a traumatic experience.

- Parasomnias may lead to psychological complications if the child is frightened, embarrassed, or otherwise upset by the experience, or because of the reactions of other people to the episodes.

13

Parasomnias when going to sleep or waking up

➡ Key points

◆ Strange experiences when drifting off to sleep or when waking up are surprisingly common in both children and adults.

◆ Although they can be alarming, they are very rarely of serious significance and almost always clear up before long.

❌ Myth versus fact

Myth: Peculiar experiences when going to sleep are unusual.

Fact: Far from it. They are, in fact, very common, including in children, who may be particularly alarmed by them but may not mention them to their parents.

Primary parasomnias when going to sleep

Sleep starts

Many parasomnias that occur when falling asleep are common and, although they may concern you, they do not mean that there is anything really wrong. Sudden, usually single, jerks of the limbs or other parts of the body when drowsy ('hypnic jerks') are particularly common. They may be accompanied by strange sensations including a feeling of falling. Less often, there may be the experience of flashes of light, a loud bang, crack or snapping noise, or another dramatic sensation. Precisely how common these experiences are at any age is not known, but they can be considered a possibility in young patients, who may be particularly alarmed by some of them. This sleep disorder should not be confused with epilepsy. Reassurance is usually all that is needed.

Hypnagogic hallucinations

Hypnagogic hallucinations may accompany sleep starts, although they often occur separately. As mentioned in Chapter 11, they can be part of the narcolepsy syndrome in which case they can be particularly intense. The far more usual and isolated form can also be frightening, consisting of a combination of a dream-like state in which objects (including people or animals) may be seen, heard, felt, smelled, tasted, or distorted, and even your own body image may seem to change. Again, these experiences, and their equivalent when waking up (hypnopompic hallucinations), do not usually mean that there is anything physically or mentally wrong.

Sleep paralysis

This condition consists of recurrent brief episodes of an inability to move or speak, either when going to sleep or when waking up, usually from a dream. You are able to move your eyes and breathe normally, yet there is often a feeling of not being able to breathe. Each episode stops of its own accord after several seconds to a minute or two, or by being touched or moved.

Sleep paralysis can also be part of the narcolepsy syndrome (see Chapter 11), but much more often it occurs by itself. Rarely, it runs in families. It appears to be common in adults and may well occur in children, although how often is not clear. The feeling of being paralysed may be accompanied by hallucinations or dream-like experiences. Understandably, all this can be very frightening, but reassurance can be given that it is not a serious condition.

Isolated sleep paralysis is likely to clear up by itself after a time.

Rhythmic movement disorder (RMD)

RMD consists of repeated movements, the same each time, mainly of the upper part of the body. The movements usually occur just before going to sleep but also after waking during the night and sometimes when waking up in the morning. The activity appears to feel pleasant for the child and may be an aid in getting to sleep or returning to sleep after waking during the night. Sometimes, these movements occur during sleep.

Headbanging is the usual type of movement, with either forward or backward impact onto a pillow or perhaps a hard surface such as the cot sides or the wall.

Head rolling and rolling or rocking movements of the whole body are other types of RMD. Combinations of these various movements can occur. The movements are often accompanied by rhythmic noises made by the child such as humming. Such episodes usually last up to 15 minutes but can be much longer.

Many children (mainly boys) have some form of sleep-related rhythmic movements in their first year of life, but the behaviour almost always stops by itself by the age of 3–4 years. Therefore, parents can be reassured that, although the behaviour may look bizarre, it is a passing phase that is not associated with any psychological or physical disorder. As in the case of sleep starts and other common experiences or behaviours when going off to sleep, RMD should not be mistaken for epilepsy.

Treatment is not usually needed except perhaps for protective measures such as padding of the cot sides. In this respect, sleep-related RMD is different from that occurring repeatedly during the day, which is often a feature of a severe developmental disorder or some other form of serious psychiatric condition such as autism. Here, the risk of head injury from headbanging is very much greater than in sleep-related headbanging.

Occasionally, more active measures are necessary for RMD because of serious disruption of the child's sleep, embarrassment, annoyance caused to others by the noise generated, or risk of injury. A number of treatments have been reported to be effective in some cases, including behavioural methods such as the use of reward systems or ways of discouraging the movements, including advising parents to avoid reinforcing the behaviour by paying too much attention to it.

Restless legs syndrome (RLS)

As many as 10% of adults complain that, especially when resting (mainly in the evening), going off to sleep, or on waking at night, they often have to move their legs (and sometimes other parts of their body) because they experience uncomfortable and unpleasant feelings. Children may well have difficulty describing these feelings, referring to them as 'creepy-crawly' sensations, for example. Walking or otherwise moving the legs may provide some relief. A high proportion of adults say their condition started when they were a child. It is thought that RLS may well be the cause of some cases of 'growing pains'.

The condition often runs in families but it can be associated with physical conditions including iron deficiency, various other medical conditions and caffeine intake, as well as certain medications such as some antidepressants.

RLS needs to be distinguished from the usual behavioural bedtime problems due to difficult behaviour or other causes of bedtime problems. Other reasons for uncomfortable legs at night include rheumatological disorders.

Most people with RLS also have frequent periodic limb movements in sleep or PLMS (see Chapter 14), but only a minority of those with PLMS also have RLS. Treatment possibilities are discussed in Chapter 14.

Primary parasomnias when waking up

The two main parasomnias experienced in this phase of sleep are hypnopompic hallucinations and sleep paralysis, both of which were described above as examples of parasomnias that can also occur at the onset of sleep.

📄 Case study

Hypnagogic hallucinations and sleep paralysis

A 20-year-old man eventually revealed that, for several years, he had experienced episodes (too embarrassing to admit to in case people thought him mad) in which, when falling asleep, he saw and heard peculiar things associated with not being able to move. Sometimes a small child would appear to him with whom he had conversations that could become heated and intimidating. Not being able to move was accompanied by a feeling that he couldn't breathe properly, which, of course, increased his anxiety considerably.

Because these experiences had become more and more frequent to the point of occurring every night, he eventually decided to see the doctor about them who arranged for him to be seen by specialists.

A psychiatrist did not think that he had the serious mental illness that had been feared. A sleep disorder specialist was then consulted who recognized the condition as a dramatic but not rare example of combined hypnagogic hallucinations and sleep paralysis.

In such cases, treatment with drugs (used in other circumstances for depression) is considered likely to be helpful. This was offered but the young man declined because he no longer thought that he was going mad.

📄 Case study

Headbanging

From the age of about 18 months, an otherwise normal boy had been banging his head repeatedly every night, initially backwards against the side of his cot and then later against the side rail of his bed while in a kneeling position. The noise of these movements, which were usually accompanied by rhythmic humming or grunting noises, disturbed the whole family. His parents thought there must be something seriously wrong with him, especially as he began to injure the skin on his forehead with the forceful banging.

As various tranquillizing and sedative drugs had been ineffective, he was seen at a paediatric sleep clinic where sleep monitoring showed that he was awake but drowsy during the rhythmic movements. A psychologist suggested a behavioural form of treatment to discourage the behaviour. This consisted of interrupting the movements by standing him up whenever they began and making him walk about, which he did not like to do. Curiously, instead, he seemed to take pleasure in banging his head. Therefore, in addition, he was praised and given a reward for not banging his head.

Within 2 weeks, the headbanging stopped. However, it recurred 6 months later at a time when financial difficulties had arisen in his family and his mother had become depressed. This affected the emotional climate of the family as a whole and made it difficult for the parents to deal effectively with the headbanging problem.

However, as soon as the family fortunes and his mother's mental state improved, his parents were able to undertake the same behavioural treatment as before, this time with lasting success.

14

Parasomnias mainly early in the night when lightly asleep

➔ Key points

◆ Some of these types of parasomnia are more common in children than was originally thought.

◆ Again, it is appropriate for the possibility of an underlying condition that requires investigation and treatment to be considered, but this will not often be the case.

❌ Myth versus fact

Myth: Odd movements (e.g. of the jaws or limbs) at the start of sleep only occur in adults.

Fact: This might once have been thought to be true, but is now known not to be the case.

Bruxism

Bruxism or teethgrinding is forceful grinding and clenching of the teeth in a paroxysmal fashion, sometimes producing a loud grinding noise at night without the person being aware. This usually occurs in light sleep, but may occur at any stage of sleep. It is thought to be particularly common in adults (although it is a serious problem in only a minority) and can be caused, for example, by stress.

Bruxism has been reported to occur in up to 20% of children, who may complain of pain in the face or a headache. In severe cases, the child's teeth might be damaged. If needed, treatment in adults may included wearing a rubber tooth guard at night if dental damage is occurring or getting psychological help if stress is a factor.

Periodic limb movements in sleep (PLMS)

PLMS are brief and stereotyped muscular contractions (usually about 2 seconds in duration) mainly affecting the toes, knees, and hips, typically every 20–40 seconds and usually without the person knowing that it is happening because he is asleep.

Very frequent PLMS are thought to be a cause of excessive daytime sleepiness in adults because they keep the person in superficial sleep, which is not as restorative as deep sleep.

PLMS can co-exist with other sleep disorders such as obstructive sleep apnoea and narcolepsy. PLMS may also be associated with iron-deficiency anaemia, various other medical disorders, the use of antidepressants, or the withdrawal of various other drugs that act on the central nervous system. PLMS are best detected by sleep recordings, which include the monitoring of limb movements.

Both PLMS and restless legs syndrome (RLS) (see Chapter 13) were thought to be rare in children and adolescents, but this now appears not to be the case, although just how often they occur at this age is not known. PLMS in particular have been implicated as a cause of daytime attention-deficit hyperactivity disorder (ADHD) symptoms, supposedly because they can cause poor-quality sleep or loss of sleep. Of the various factors that can underlie sleep disturbance in children with a learning difficulty, PLMS have been particularly implicated in some specific syndromes.

Conditions somewhat clinically similar to RLS include muscle cramps, disorders of the peripheral nerves, and certain muscle disorders.

The effectiveness of the various reported treatments for both RLS and PLMS (which are best limited to those who are prevented from sleeping well or who are excessively sleepy during the day or have other daytime problems convincingly caused by these sleep disorders) appears to be variable in adults. As there is little information about these treatments in children, emphasis should be placed on good sleep hygiene, although medication may be justified in some cases.

In the case of RLS, some benefit may be gained from avoiding caffeine in particular, taking iron supplements where necessary, undertaking moderate exercise in the evening, and, because of the link with inactivity, not going to bed until ready to sleep rather than lying in bed awake.

15

Parasomnias when deeply asleep: 'arousal disorders'

➔ Key points

- These sleep disorders (which include sleepwalking) are common in children, who usually grow out of them before adulthood.

- The tendency to have these disorders is often inherited.

- Some can be alarming for parents to witness, but, as the child remains asleep during the episodes, he himself will not actually be distressed.

- There can be a risk, however, that the child will be accidentally injured.

- Parents need to know what to do and what not to do when these episodes occur.

✖ Myth versus fact

Myth: Sleepwalking is unusual.

Fact: It is actually quite common.

Myth: A child who seems frightened when sleepwalking or having a sleep terror should be woken up and comforted by his parents.

Fact: This is what not to do. The child may appear to be frightened but actually isn't because he is asleep. If he is forcefully woken, he will be confused and upset.

Disorders of arousal (i.e. confusional arousals, sleepwalking, and sleep terrors) are very common in childhood. In a minority of people, they persist into adult life, whilst in a few they begin in adolescence.

Arousal does not mean that the child wakes up; the arousal is, in fact, a 'partial arousal', usually from deep non-rapid eye movement (NREM) sleep (slow wave sleep or SWS) to another lighter stage of sleep. In such arousals, various behaviours can occur that are either simple in nature (for example, sitting up in bed and mumbling) or more complicated, such as rushing out of the house in a highly agitated state. Other, complex behaviours occasionally described in young people include aggressive acts and sleep-related eating disorders.

It is important to realise that the child remains asleep during the arousal episode itself and therefore fails to recognize his parents or be comforted by them, although waking sometimes occurs at the end of the episode, particularly in later childhood or adolescence.

Usually only one episode occurs during the night, within the first 2 hours or so after going to sleep when SWS is most abundant. Rarely, multiple episodes occur throughout the night, in which case each episode is usually less dramatic than the previous one. Partial arousals are possible during daytime naps.

The tendency to have an arousal disorder is basically inherited: a child with this type of sleep disorder is likely to have a close blood relative with the same type of condition. Children and adolescents with this predisposition may have their attacks precipitated by

- fever or other illness;

- sedative medication and possibly alcohol;

- interruption of their sleep, e.g. by a full bladder, a sudden loud noise, or other sleep disorders such as obstructive sleep apnoea;

- sleeping in an unfamiliar environment;

- stress.

The more dramatic forms of arousal disorder in particular may well be thought by parents to mean that their child has a psychiatric disorder, but this is rarely so. However, arousal disorders can be embarrassing and emotionally upsetting, especially when they occur away from home.

As in other parasomnias, the main way of recognizing arousal disorders is to compile a detailed description of what happens in the episodes, ideally from their very beginning right the way through until your child is his usual self again. A home video system (preferably with sound) can be extremely valuable in helping to achieve this. Only in particularly difficult cases will physiological sleep studies (polysomnography) be needed.

Types of arousal disorder

There are three types of arousal disorder:

- confusional arousals;

- sleepwalking;

- sleep terrors.

All have in common a curious combination of features suggestive of being awake and asleep at the same time. Despite seeming to be alert (and indeed sometimes highly aroused), because he is actually asleep, the child appears confused, disoriented, and relatively unresponsive to his environment, including his parents' attempts to communicate with him. There is little or (usually) no memory of what happened during each episode.

A child might have confusional arousals in early childhood, developing into sleepwalking later, followed by sleep terrors in late childhood and adolescence. Alternatively, elements of all three forms can occur at any one stage of development. Similarly, arousal disorders in other family members can take various forms.

Confusional arousals

These occur mainly in infants and toddlers. An episode may begin with movements and moaning and then progress to agitated and confused behaviour with crying (perhaps intense), calling out, or thrashing about. Typically, although appearing very alert, the child does not respond when spoken to.

Parents are often alarmed and, wanting to console their child, they may make vigorous attempts to waken him, without success or only managing after much trying. However, such efforts may actually prolong the arousal and, if the child is woken to some extent, he is likely to be confused and frightened.

Each episode usually lasts 5–15 minutes (possibly longer) before the child calms down spontaneously and begins to sleep quietly again.

Sleepwalking

Sleepwalking (or 'somnambulism') occurs occasionally in 20–40% of children and frequently in another 3–4%, mainly between the ages of 4 and 8.

Episodes, lasting up to 10 minutes or so, are usually less dramatic than confusional arousals. The young child may crawl or walk about in his cot. At a later age, he may calmly walk around his room or into other parts of the house such as to the toilet, towards a light, or to his parents' bedroom. The child may appear downstairs or may be found standing on the landing or elsewhere in the house, looking vague, with eyes open but with a glassy stare. At most, he will be partially responsive. Some children are found asleep in various parts of the house. Quite complicated routes may be followed if they are well known to the child, or other complex habitual behaviour (automatism) may occur, possibly lasting for long periods of time. The child's movements are often clumsy. Urinating in inappropriate places or other confused behaviour is common.

There is a serious risk of accidental injury in sleepwalking (e.g. from falling downstairs). In later childhood or adolescence, the wandering may extend further within the house or outside it. At this age and later, the sleepwalking may take an agitated form (similar to sleep terrors), which may be worsened by attempts to intervene and with an even greater risk of injury from crashing through windows or glass doors, for example.

Sleep terrors

'Night terrors' (sometimes referred to as *pavor nocturnus*) are better called sleep terrors as they are associated with sleep, whenever it may occur. They are reported in about 3% of children, mainly in later childhood.

Typically, parents are woken by their child's piercing scream at the sudden start of the sleep terror. They then find him apparently terrified, with staring eyes, profuse sweating, a rapid pulse, and crying out as if intensely distressed. He may jump out of bed and rush about frantically, as if trying to escape from something. Inevitably, injury caused by running into furniture or jumping through windows is a serious risk, as in agitated sleepwalking. The event usually lasts no more than a few minutes at most.

Generally, the episode ends abruptly and the child settles back to sleep. If he wakes up at the end of the episode, he may describe feelings of primitive threat or danger, but not a nightmare (see Chapter 16).

Advice and treatment for arousal disorders

Parents' anxieties are usually lessened by an explanation together with reassurance (where justified) that these sometimes dramatic and alarming events do not mean that their child is ill or emotionally disturbed, and that usually he can be expected to grow out of them by later childhood or adolescence.

Regular and adequate sleep routines to prevent loss or disruption of sleep resulting in an increased amount of SWS are important, as well as avoiding as far as possible other factors that have been observed to precipitate arousal disorder episodes.

The child's environment should be made as safe as possible to reduce the risk of injury, for example by the removal of obstructions in the bedroom, securing windows, installing locks or alarms on outside doors, and covering windows with heavy curtains.

Attempts by parents to waken their child or restrain him during the episode are not appropriate and can do more harm than good. Waking the child is likely to be difficult and, if achieved abruptly, will result in him feeling confused and frightened—quite the opposite of what his parents are aiming to do in their attempt to console him. It is also unnecessary. It is much better to wait until the episode subsides and calmly help the child back to bed.

If, as is usually the case, the child does not know about the episode, because he was asleep when it happened, there is little point in telling him about it, as this may make him anxious about himself.

If sleepwalking or sleep terror episodes are frequent and consistent in the time at which they occur, 'scheduled awakening' might be helpful. This consists of the child being gently and briefly woken about 15 minutes before the episode is due. The procedure is repeated nightly for up to 1 month.

Medication, such as benzodiazepines, should be reserved for particularly worrying, embarrassing, or dangerous arousals where other measures have failed. Use of a benzodiazepine drug (such as a small dose of clonazepam) should usually be limited to several weeks at most to avoid the possible hazards of long-term use.

If there is evidence of an underlying psychological problem, appropriate enquiries should be arranged.

📄 Case study

Sleepwalking

Late one evening, the parents of a 5-year-old girl heard a crash and then someone crying intensely at the rear of their house. They went outside to find her lying on the patio under her open first-floor bedroom window. She had fallen out of the window and was lying face down with both of her wrists broken.

For the past 2 years, the girl had suffered from sleepwalking episodes inside the house (a tendency that she shared with her brother and also her father when he was young), but she had not previously come to any harm.

Her parents were sure that the window through which she had fallen was always securely fastened. To have opened it, the girl must have climbed on to a chest of drawers, slid the inner double-glazing sideways and then unfastened the window catch before swinging the window open and climbing through.

Not knowing that such complicated behaviour was possible while still asleep, they were at a loss to know what could have happened and wondered if she had climbed through the window on purpose. However, there was no reason at all why she would have done such a thing. The staff at the hospital to which she was taken were equally confused about what had really happened. The girl herself said that she could remember nothing between going to sleep and finding herself on the ground in pain.

Subsequently, the incident was reviewed including advice from a child psychiatrist in case there may after all have been some psychological reason for the girl's behaviour. However, there still did not appear to be any evidence of this. More to the point, the psychiatrist emphasized that some sleepwalkers do indeed perform very complicated acts while still asleep.

This being so, taken with the girl's past history of sleepwalking, the fact that her injury seemed to have occurred within about 2 hours of her going to sleep, and that she had no memory of climbing through the window, he was confident that the accident had occurred during a sleepwalking episode.

A programme of treatment was devised including taking various safety measures and a scheduled awakening procedure (see above).

16

Parasomnias mainly later in the night

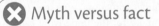

→ Key points

♦ Parasomnias that mainly occur later in the night are likely to be linked to rapid eye movement (REM) sleep.

♦ True nightmares have specific identifiable features and should not be confused with other, different dramatic parasomnias for which the term 'nightmare' is sometimes loosely used.

✖ Myth versus fact

Myth: Nightmares are a sign of an emotional problem.

Fact: This is not usually the case. Many people, including children, have an occasional nightmare without this being of serious significance.

Nightmares

Nightmares (i.e. frightening dreams that wake you up, as distinct from disturbing dreams without waking) are the obvious example of a parasomnia related to REM (or 'dreaming') sleep. Unfortunately, the term 'nightmare' is sometimes loosely used for any type of dramatic night-time episode.

True nightmares, which typically occur in the later part of overnight sleep when most REM sleep is present, occur in up to 75% of children from early childhood onwards. The frightening content of the dream varies with the child's age, tending to become increasingly complex; for example, monsters and other frightening creatures at an early age, progressing to dreams based on frightening TV or film content or events at home or school.

Typically, your child wakes up, alarmed and fully alert, and describes having just had a frightening, vividly recalled dream, often involving the child himself. He remains afraid after waking and cannot get back to sleep for some time, although it is usually possible to reassure and comfort him.

Nightmares may occur for no clear reason or (like arousal disorders) they can be precipitated by illness or psychological stress. Generally, such dreams are infrequent without any serious psychological significance. However, particularly frequent nightmares may well be part of an anxiety disorder including post-traumatic stress disorder, and their content, especially if consistent, may reflect the nature of the traumatic experience. In such circumstances, nightmares may be accompanied by bedtime fears.

Usually, there is nothing more that needs to be done at the time other than comforting your child when the nightmare occurs. Avoiding disturbing stories or videos before going to bed and other sources of overexcitement or distress might well help to prevent nightmares occurring.

In severe cases, and with professional advice, helping the child to be less concerned about the frightening content of the nightmare, or rehearsing the content but with a modified, less alarming ending, is sometimes effective. In even more complicated cases, psychological treatment for the underlying cause of the nightmare may be needed.

REM sleep behaviour disorder (RBD)

This is a relatively newly described parasomnia that used to be thought to be a condition only in elderly men. However, it (or a similar disorder) has now been reported in other groups, including women and (rarely) in children.

Normally you are paralysed in REM sleep and are unable to act out your dreams; however, people with RBD are not paralysed in this way and therefore they can act out their dreams and may, if they have violent dreams, behave violently, such as punching, kicking, leaping, or running about, often causing self-injury or injury to anyone nearby.

In adults, RBD is often associated with various neurological disorders and some medications, but there is often no obvious cause although the underlying disorder may develop in time. The same is true of the relatively few children with this condition. Because of its strong associations with organic factors, RBD is often considered one of the secondary parasomnias (see Chapter 12).

RBD is recognized by the strange behaviour and, using special sleep studies, the REM sleep abnormality described above. Clonazepam is usually an effective treatment.

📄 **Case study**

Nightmares

A 6-year-old girl had been perfectly well with no sleep problems until soon after the family pet dog, to which she was very attached, died. On average about once a week, she began to wake up late in the night in a highly agitated state, usually crying profusely. She was able to describe that she had been having a complicated dream that ended by her pet dog being run over by a car (as had actually happened) and being in pain. At other times, the dream was about herself being lost somewhere strange, being pursued by some sort of animal, and not being able to get back home to her parents.

During these dream experiences, she became increasingly upset to the point of suddenly waking up and crying out for her parents. When they went to her room, they would find her in a distressed state but fully alert and aware of her surroundings. They were able to comfort her with hugs and reassurances that she had been having a frightening dream and that she was perfectly safe, although it could sometimes take many minutes before she was able to relax and go back to sleep.

It seemed that the loss of her pet dog had brought on the nightmares rather than any other upsetting circumstances in her life calling for special help. The family doctor's advice to her parents was to continue to handle further nightmares in the same way as they had already done, avoiding transmitting any anxiety that they themselves might feel at their child being so upset, and to encourage her to reassure herself that it was only a dream next time she had a nightmare. Other suggestions were to avoid frightening TV programmes or stories before bedtime, to ensure that she had enough sleep, to have a comfort object with her in bed (such as her favourite doll), and also to use a dim nightlight in her bedroom.

In case the nightmares became more severe and frequent, additional possible measures were mentioned to be tried with the guidance of a child psychologist. These included relaxation treatments or ways of gradually removing the fear element of the frightening components of her nightmares ('systematic desensitization') or practising imagining positive alternative endings to her nightmare experiences. Fortunately, these approaches proved unnecessary as, in a matter of 3–4 weeks, the nightmares became less frequent and stopped completely after a further month.

17

Parasomnias that occur at various times of the night

> ## ➲ Key points
>
> ◆ Some of the strange or troublesome behaviours related to sleep are not as tied to particular stages of sleep as other parasomnias.
>
> ◆ Their significance and the advice or treatment they require varies.

> ## ✖ Myth versus fact
>
> **Myth:** Talking in your sleep means that you have something troubling you on your mind.
>
> **Fact:** This is unlikely to be true. Most sleep talking, in itself, is of no significance.
>
> **Myth:** Children who wet the bed are emotionally disturbed.
>
> **Fact:** This can be the case, but more usually there is another explanation for it, although the child (and his parents) may get upset as a result of frequent wet beds.

Sleep talking

Sleep talking is common and can occur by itself or as a part of various sleep disorders such as arousal disorder, obstructive sleep apnoea, or REM sleep behaviour disorder, and in all phases of sleep. Some people talk in their sleep for no apparent reason or in response to being talked to. It is usually brief and does not make much sense. Often, it consists mainly of moaning noises.

By itself, sleep talking is of no real significance apart from the annoyance caused to others trying to sleep nearby. Treatment is only possible if there is a particular underlying sleep disorder.

Nocturnal enuresis (bedwetting)

Nocturnal enuresis is a particularly common problem in children. It is officially defined as recurrent involuntary bedwetting in the absence of a physical cause in a child over the age of 5 years. Bedwetting at least once a week occurs in about 5% of 7-year-olds and 3% of 9-year-olds. Around 2% are still affected at the age 11 and perhaps 1% by 14 years of age or older. Boys increasingly outnumber girls as the age of the child increases. Enuresis tends to happen early in sleep, but can occur at any stage of sleep.

Children are said to have 'primary enuresis' if they have never been able to control their bladder (70–90% of cases); 'secondary enuresis' means loss of control after acquiring it for at least 3 months.

The main possible causes of primary nocturnal enuresis are:

* delayed maturation of bladder mechanisms (possibly genetic, as it is often seen in other family members);

* possibly limited bladder capacity but (more likely) feeling the need to empty the bladder before it is full more readily than most children;

* failure to toilet-train the child satisfactorily;

* general delay in a child's development.

Secondary nocturnal enuresis (which may be accompanied by wetting during the day) can be caused by physical factors such as:

* a urinary tract infection (especially girls);

* anatomical abnormalities of the urinary tract;

* medical conditions that cause overproduction of urine (e.g. diabetes);

* pressure on the bladder by, for example, a faecal mass in chronic constipation;

* obstructive sleep apnoea;

- nocturnal epilepsy;

- some spinal deformities;

- possibly some allergies.

However, in addition, it may be associated with:

- emotional upset (e.g. starting a new school, the arrival of a new baby, or, more seriously, abuse or neglect);

- arousal disorders such as sleepwalking.

Nocturnal enuresis is likely to result in embarrassment and upset for the child (restricting social activities away from home), as well as annoying parents who may become less than sympathetic to their child.

The following points about treatment are worth bearing in mind if you child suffers from nocturnal enuresis.

- Clearly, primary and secondary enuresis have to be distinguished from each other as the investigations and treatment required will be very different. Your doctor will arrange the necessary investigations if there is evidence of secondary enuresis.

- Making the child feel guilty, as if the bedwetting is his fault, and punishment and expression of disappointment must be avoided at all costs.

- Instead, reassurance, rewards for dry nights, and a positive attitude are required.

- Restricting fluids before bedtime or waking your child to go to the toilet before you go to bed or during the night tend to be unhelpful.

- Conditioning by use of an alarm system (such as the 'pad and bell' procedure, which aims to form an association between having the sensation of a full bladder and waking up to go to the toilet) can be effective if attempted in a systematic, consistent, and determined way. This entirely safe procedure involves the child lying on a pad or wearing it inside his pyjamas; as he begins to wet himself, the wet pad forms an electrical connection to an alarm that wakes him up.

- Medication should be considered if other treatments have not worked, e.g. desmopressin for short-term use or for special circumstances, such as when staying with friends for a brief period. Some drugs that used in other circumstances to treat depression have also been used but may be less effective.

- ◆ Bladder training during the day to increase bladder capacity and stability is another measure that has been used successfully.

- ◆ Various treatments may sometimes be used in combination.

- ◆ The time taken for treatment to be effective can vary significantly from one child to another and relapses also may occur, calling for the treatment to be started again.

- ◆ Psychiatric help should be provided in the few cases where this is appropriate.

- ◆ In the case of primary enuresis in particular, it should be remembered that the problem may well clear up of its own accord, given time.

📄 Case study

Bedwetting

Much to his dismay (and also his parents' consternation), a 7-year-old boy was still wetting his bed most nights, having done so all of his life. This was embarrassing to him and prevented him staying overnight with friends. His younger brother, with whom he shared his bedroom, was only too aware of the problem and made matters worse by making fun of him.

The bedwetting was a problem for his mother in particular because of constantly having to change his pyjamas and bed sheets and wash them. Fortunately, he only wet himself at night and not at all during the day. His father was sympathetic because he had wet the bed as a child and had also been embarrassed until eventually it stopped without any treatment.

The boy was otherwise healthy and doing quite well at school, although his parents thought he was more than usually shy in company. He did not appear to be unduly anxious or depressed, but eventually he himself asked if he should see the doctor about wetting the bed. Until then, his parents had not sought help, hoping that he would soon become dry as his father had done. However, the problem seemed to be taking longer and, in the meantime, the family atmosphere was becoming fraught.

Their GP referred him to a local child psychologist who recognized the bedwetting as primary enuresis that did not need to be investigated medically. She told the boy that his was a common problem and was not his fault in any way, and that, given time, it would clear up although there were ways of speeding up the process. Whilst understanding his mother's feelings in particular, she emphasized the importance of being sympathetic and avoiding making him feel guilty. She also suggested that the parents discourage their other son from making fun of him, explaining that this only made things worse.

This advice improved the emotional climate within the family and the bedwetting became less frequent. The GP prescribed a short course of desmopressin for when the boy stayed at a friend's house overnight and when he went on a week's camping trip with the school. This also helped to make him feel better about himself.

However, as he was still wetting the bed about once every 10 days or so, she recommended the use of a bell and pad system every night to help the boy learn to associate the feeling of a full bladder with the need to wake up and go to the toilet. Having had the procedure explained to him, he accepted it quite happily. Combined with being rewarded for dry nights, this seemed to work more readily than it usually does in other children and, after about 6 weeks, he became dry and remained so when he stopped using the pad and bell apparatus.

18

Unusual behaviour at night associated with medical conditions

→ Key points

◆ Although not usually the case, there are some parasomnias that result from an underlying medical condition; these need to be distinguished from other parasomnias.

◆ Treatment consists of attention to the underlying condition.

◆ The distinction between medically based and other parasomnias can often be made by knowing the exact nature of the episodes, but in some instances special investigations are required.

✕ Myth versus fact

Myth: Strange behaviour at night is due to psychological problems that require psychological help.

Fact: This can be the case but is unusual. Often the episodes are undoubtedly medical in nature.

Myth: Epilepsy means having convulsions.

Fact: A convulsion is only one of many types of epileptic attack. Other types include seizures which involve unusual behaviour or being very disturbed. If these occur at night, they might well be mistaken for other types of non-epileptic sleep disorders such as sleep terrors.

Examples have been given in previous chapters of how sleep can be disturbed in various ways in a number of medical and psychological disorders. Parasomnias illustrate this point very well.

Epilepsies associated with sleep

There are many types of epilepsy, which different from each other in their cause, type of attack, effects, treatment needs, and outlook for the future. A number of these types are closely related to the sleep–wake cycle including the following, which can easily be confused with non-epileptic parasomnias.

Benign partial epilepsy with centro-temporal spikes (Rolandic epilepsy)

This complicated-sounding condition is, in fact, is a common form of child-hood epilepsy in which about 75% of patients have their attacks (or 'seizures') only when they are asleep. During the seizure, the child usually experiences strange feelings in his mouth and face, which can be very frightening.

The seizures occur when falling asleep, in the middle of the night or (most commonly) when waking up. The condition is diagnosed mainly from the distinctive features of the seizure described above, helped by a characteristic findings on an electroencephalogram or EEG (brain wave test).

It is important that these seizures are not mistaken for other forms of epilepsy or different types of parasomnia such as sleep terrors. Despite their frightening nature, they are not a sign of any serious brain disease and stop of their own accord, usually after a few years. Medication is not usually required.

Nocturnal frontal lobe epilepsy

This form of epilepsy, which occurs in both adults and children, can be mistaken for a psychological disorder because the seizures often involve strange movements (e.g. kicking, hitting, rocking, thrashing, and cycling, or scissor movements of the legs) and noises (from grunting, coughing, muttering, or moaning to shouting, screaming, or roaring).

Again, the distinctive nature of the seizures in this form of epilepsy should help to avoid a wrong diagnosis. In contrast to the condition described above, EEG findings may well be unhelpful. The underlying cause varies although one form is clearly inherited. Response to treatment is also variable.

Other epilepsies associated with sleep

Various other types of childhood epilepsy, in which the seizures arise in different parts of the brain including the temporal lobes, may well have features in common with some of the more dramatic types of primary parasomnia, at least in older children. This is particularly so where fear is a prominent feature, either as part of the seizure itself or as a reaction to the strange experiences involved.

Obviously, the distinction between epilepsy and other parasomnias is essential. This should be possible in most cases by a careful description of the child's attacks, combined with the appropriate special investigations.

Epilepsy can interact with other sleep disorders. For example, seizures can occur more frequently if a child also has obstructive sleep apnoea, in which case the epilepsy may well improve when the sleep apnoea is treated.

Other parasomnias of medical origin

Examples of these in both adults and children include:

- some forms of migraine that can include odd experiences;

- fearful awakenings caused by respiratory disorders such as asthma or obstructive sleep apnoea;

- restless legs syndrome and periodic limb movements in sleep (both of which can be symptomatic of an underlying physical illness; see Chapters 13 and 14);

- REM sleep behaviour disorder (see Chapter 16), which may well be secondary to neurological disease or medication.

Case study

Night-time epileptic attacks

Advice was requested from a sleep disorders clinic about a 10-year-old girl who a year before, having previously been perfectly well, had began to have episodes of very disturbed behaviour at various times during the night.

As part of the initial assessment, and at the suggestion of the clinic, her parents videoed several of the episodes using their own video system.

This, and her parents' observations when they went to her room, showed that the episodes were all basically the same. Each began with her suddenly sitting up in bed looking very frightened and crying out, sweating profusely, and having a flushed face. She then began rushing about her bedroom, as if being pursued, before cowering in a corner whimpering and unresponsive to her parents' attempts to comfort her. After about 2 minutes at most, she calmed down quite rapidly and could be put back to bed where she fell sound asleep again.

When first consulted, her doctor thought that she might be suffering from sleep terrors, but there were several points against this diagnosis. She had no past history of any arousal disorder and no family history of this type of condition; also, the episodes did not tend to occur in the first part of the night. More to the point, the episodes had become increasingly frequent so that they were happening as often as 20 times a night, throughout the night.

Reassessment in the sleep disorders centre included overnight sleep recordings during the episodes with special emphasis on EEG activity, as well as special brain imaging studies. The main finding was that the attacks were epileptic in nature (seeming to arise in one temporal part of the brain) but with no evidence of any anatomical abnormality to account for them. There was nothing to suggest any additional parasomnia of the various types that involve dramatic night-time disturbance.

The findings were carefully explained to the girl and her parents. She was treated successfully with anti-epileptic medication and her progress was followed up carefully.

19

Psychiatric disorders that cause unusual behaviour at night

➜ Key points

◆ Accurate assessment and the application of specific treatment are also important here, as in the case of parasomnias that are part of a medical condition.

✖ Myth versus fact

Myth: Strange night-time behaviour means that a child is psychologically disturbed.

Fact: The point was made at the start of the last chapter that parasomnias can sometimes be part of a psychological disorder, although this is by no means often the case. Nevertheless, it is important for such problems are correctly identified so that appropriate help can be given, preferably at an early stage.

Disturbances of behaviour or experience may occur in certain psychiatric or behavioural disorders for which psychological help is needed, rather than attention to the sleep disorder alone.

Nightmares are acknowledged to be a prominent feature of post-traumatic stress disorder, which is associated with various traumatic experiences in childhood or adult life.

Nocturnal panic attacks in children and adolescents may not be recognized as such because of the features they share with other causes of apparently fearful behaviour at night, such as nightmares, night terrors, obstructive sleep apnoea awakenings, and some seizures. In a night-time panic attack, the child suddenly wakes up in a highly aroused state with dizziness, choking, sweating, trembling, palpitations, and other distressing sensations, including an intense fear of 'impending doom' (e.g. of dying). The same sort of attacks may or may not also occur during the day. Various ways of reducing anxiety can helpful, including behavioural treatment and medication.

Sleep-related eating disorder is mainly a problem in adult females, but the often bizarre eating practices at night may begin in childhood. There may be an abnormal eating pattern during the day. The night-time behaviour is mainly linked to sleepwalking, but may also occur in people with obstructive sleep apnoea, restless legs syndrome, narcolepsy, or other causes of disrupted sleep. Treatment involves treatment of the underlying sleep disorder.

In so-called **dissociative states**, people behave in ways of which, for psychological reasons, they are unaware. Dramatic behaviour (sometimes bizarre or violent) may occur at night-time while awake. Some people seem to start behaving in this fashion in later childhood or adolescence.

This last condition may be difficult to distinguish from **malingering**, where someone (occasionally a young person) is fully aware of what he is doing and why—for example, to gain attention. The person may pretend to have epileptic attacks while asleep or other parasomnias when actually he is awake, as can be shown if sleep recordings are taken at the time. Clearly, the reason for behaving in this way needs to be discovered, so that appropriate psychological help can be provided.

📄 Case study

Panic attacks

A 16-year-old girl eventually told her parents that, starting about 6 months earlier, she had increasingly experienced episodes at night, after being asleep for 2–3 hours, of suddenly waking up in a state of intense panic.

Previously, for about a year, this sort of thing had happened during the day under various circumstances for no apparent reason. Typically, when this happened, she felt an compelling need to escape from wherever she was at the time. This was often difficult because she was still attending school. To the increasing concern of her parents and teachers, she had to stop whatever she was doing and go somewhere quiet to recover over a period of half an hour or so.

Her GP arranged for her to be seen again at the local adolescent psychiatry clinic where it was decided that her panic attacks were another sign of an anxiety disorder for which she had previously attended the clinic. It was thought that she shared with her mother a tendency to be anxious as part of her general make-up, rather than because of any particular traumatic experience. The question now arose as to whether her new night-time episodes were another part of this tendency or were some other sleep disorder.

Apart from the time at which they occurred, her day-time and night-time attacks showed identical features. In both, she suddenly became very highly aroused and intensely fearful that she was going to die, and these feelings were associated with dizziness, sweating, trembling, palpitations, rapid breathing, and a feeling that she was suffocating. Afterwards, she remembered these experiences vividly. After about 10 minutes, she was able to calm down but usually had difficulty getting back to sleep.

She was not taking any medication that might have disturbed her sleep in this way and, following careful assessment, no evidence was found that she was suffering from any of the other parasomnias that can cause or suggest intense distress such as sleep terrors, some forms of epilepsy, or obstructive sleep apnoea. As described above, there was no reason to suspect that her sleep disturbance was part of a post-traumatic stress disorder and there was no doubt at all that her distress was genuine.

It was explained to the girl and her parents that her night-time attacks were simply a part of her tendency to be anxious and were not some additional type of disorder, and that it should be possible to treat these attacks. The treatment that she was already taking for her general anxiety condition (a combination of behavioural measures and medication) was increased. In time, both her daytime and night-time panic attacks became much less frequent and her overall anxiety levels also improved.

20

Children at high risk of sleep disorders

→ Key points

◆ Some groups of children are at particular risk of sleep problems that can be serious and complicated.

◆ They can often be helped providing the cause of their sleep disturbance is correctly identified and appropriate treatment is given.

✖ Myth versus fact

Myth: The sleep problems of children with developmental disorders, such as learning disabilities, are usually not possible to treat.

Fact: This is not so. The same treatment methods that are used for other children are appropriate and are likely to be effective if used correctly.

It was mentioned in Chapter 2 that, however common sleep problems are in children in general, they occur much more often in certain subgroups. It is worth enlarging on this because it is a serious matter if sleep disturbance is added to the problems already faced by such children and their families.

The following points are worth emphasizing.

◆ These 'high-risk' children do not have a different set of sleep problems and disorders compared with other children. It is simply that the frequency and pattern of occurrence is different.

◆ Often, they have a combination of 'behavioural' sleep problems (from not having acquired good sleep habits) and those of a medical or psychiatric sort, reflecting the nature of their basic condition. Both types of problem need to be treated but in different ways.

◆ In so far as it is possible, the underlying illness or disorder should, of course, be treated.

◆ The response to a correctly chosen and properly implemented treatment for the sleep disorder itself can be as good in these high-risk children as in other children.

Chronic physical illness, disorder, or disability

Just about any acute illness can affect your child's sleep but only for the duration of the illness, which is usually short. However, if he has to be admitted to hospital, this in itself will probably disturb his sleep patterns and this may continue for some time after his return home.

The main difficulties arise with long-term (chronic) health problems. In fact, it is hard to think of an example where sleep is unlikely to be affected. This should not be overlooked by preoccupation with the physical aspects of the condition itself. The effects of the sleep problem are likely to add significantly to the difficulties in coping with the basic underlying condition.

Sleep may be disturbed by physical conditions in various ways.

◆ **Discomfort or pain** accompanies many illnesses or disorders such as severe skin complaints, arthritis, malignancies, and burns. Some children with cerebral palsy or neuromuscular disease, for example, cannot get comfortable in bed or reposition themselves at night, causing them enough discomfort to disrupt their sleep.

◆ **Some conditions get worse at night**. In Chapter 18, some forms of epilepsy that occur mainly (if not exclusively) at night were described. Asthmatic attacks sometimes also worsen during sleep.

◆ **Obstructive sleep apnoea and similar breathing problems** frequently occur in various types of learning disability such as Down syndrome, some forms of cerebral palsy, neuromuscular disorders, and other neurological disorders, as well as head and facial deformities in which breathing during sleep is made difficult because of obstruction of the upper airways. The increasing problem of childhood obesity also causes breathing problems in sleep.

- **Sensory impairment** can upset sleep in different ways. Children who have been blind since birth are deprived of light perception, which is the main way by which the body clock (see Chapter 1) organizes the sleep–wake cycle. As a result, the sleep pattern of such children is likely to be disorganized, although melatonin can be used to help with this. Lesser degrees of visual impairment will not have such direct serious effects on sleep. Here, sleep problems are more likely to be behavioural in nature. Profoundly deaf children may also have abnormal sleep patterns, and those with tinnitus (ringing in the ears) may be disturbed at night when they become more aware of it in the quietness of night.

- **Other forms of chronic illness** such as endocrine, kidney, or liver disease can upset sleep mechanisms because of a general disturbance of bodily functions. Children with severe head injury often have various sleep problems, partly depending on which part of the brain is mainly damaged. The same can be true of children with brain tumours.

- Some types of **medication** for children's physical ailments can upset sleep. For example, some drugs that help breathing can cause sleeplessness.

📄 Case study

Visual impairment

The sleep pattern of a 2-year-old girl who had been blind from birth because of severe brain abnormalities was said to be very variable in how long she slept and when. Sometimes she was awake all night and asleep all day. Sleeping medicine did not work and her mother described herself as 'at her wits' end'.

The results of a sleep diary completed over a 4-week period confirmed that the child's sleep was indeed highly disorganized, usually with frequent daytime naps at irregular times, and that her night-time sleep was also broken into several short periods. She attended a nursery but was often too tired to join in the activities.

The first attempts to produce a more regular sleep–wake pattern consisted of encouraging a highly regular routine for sleeping, meals, and all other activities, including interaction with other people (especially her mother), and making as much use as possible of non-visual cues as to whether it was day or night. This helped to confine her sleep mainly to night-time. Melatonin was taken before bedtime, which helped matters further.

Learning disability (mental retardation or intellectual disability)

As these terms cover a wide range of conditions that differ considerably in their cause, severity, and associated problems, general statements about sleep problems in children with such limited ability are bound to be misleading in some cases. However, parents often report that their children have difficulties with their sleep, and that these difficulties are often severe and persistent. Many such problems are behavioural in origin, for example because the child has not learnt good sleep habits, perhaps because of his parents' reluctance to teach him or because they (mistakenly) have assumed it would not work even if they tried. This would only be likely in the relatively few children whose learning disability is the result of particularly severe brain damage in which sleep mechanisms have not developed or have been put out of action.

Children with a learning disability may have associated medical disorders that affect their sleep and that call for attention in their own right. The common occurrence of obstructive sleep apnoea has already been mentioned. Epilepsy may also be a complicating factor, especially if seizures occur frequently at night. Sleep can be expected to improve with better seizure control. Fortunately, modern anti-epileptic medication does not usually upset sleep or make a child sleepy during the day.

A child with a learning disability may have one or more of the other sleep-disturbing neurological problems mentioned in Chapter 18.

Case study

Learning disability

Because of serious complications when she was born, a 3-year-old girl was quite severely impaired intellectually and also suffered from epilepsy and the spastic form of cerebral palsy. Her parents said that she had always cried a lot at night, but that recently this had become worse and, in addition, she now woke repeatedly feeling distressed and wanting them to be with her.

Her parents had developed the practice of letting her go to sleep downstairs in their arms and then allowing her to sleep in their own bed every night where she awoke every hour or two and needed much comforting before she settled back to sleep again. Most of her infrequent seizures occurred during the day, consisting of being unresponsive for a few seconds. At night, she had occasional episodes of stiffening for a matter of several seconds, which were thought to be another type of seizure.

Overall, she obtained about 7 hours of sleep a night compared with the average of about 12 hours required for children of her age. She did not sleep excessively during the day and was described as generally miserable and difficult to manage.

Her only treatment was medication for her cerebral palsy. Anti-epileptic medication had not been used because her seizures were infrequent and mild. Sleeping medicine had been tried at times but had not worked and possibly had made her more irritable during the day.

The advice at the paediatric unit that she attended was to concentrate on teaching her better sleep habits because, in her case (unlike some other children with multiple conditions), the epilepsy and cerebral palsy were not likely to be disturbing her sleep. The main aim was to try to reduce her need for her parents to be with her at bedtime and to get back to sleep when she awoke in the night.

The behavioural ways of achieving this (described in Chapters 4 and 5) were used, initially with limited success because her parents felt unable to change their habits and, where necessary, to be firm but gentle in carrying out the procedures. However, with support and encouragement from the unit staff, they were eventually able to do what was required. After a matter of some weeks, their daughter's settling and night-waking problems improved considerably and she appeared to be more contented during the day.

Psychiatric problems

Just as it is difficult to point to any serious medical disorder that in not usually complicated by disturbed sleep, the same is true of psychiatric conditions. A particular difficulty, however, can be to know which came first—the psychiatric problem or the sleep disturbance—because, as discussed in Chapter 2, loss of sleep or poor-quality sleep can upset behaviour in many ways, sometimes seriously. For example, reference has been made at several points to a sleep disorder being the cause of some cases of attention-deficit hyperactivity disorder (ADHD) and depression can also be brought on by not sleeping well.

Ideally, the conundrum can be solved by looking back to see whether the sleep problem developed before the psychiatric problem, or the other way round. Given this information, many examples come to light where the sleep disturbance is a feature of the psychiatric disorder, such as the parasomnias described in Chapter 19. Other examples are as follows.

- People with **depressive disorders**, including children and adolescents, often have difficulty getting to sleep or staying asleep. Many depressed adolescents complain that they are very sleepy during the day in a way that may not only be the result of not sleeping well at night. A variation on this theme is seen in children with seasonal affective disorder or SAD (see Chapter 11).

- Children who are **anxious** have difficulty getting to sleep and also have broken sleep, and sometimes also nightmares (as part of post-traumatic stress disorder), night-time panic attacks, and sleepwalking, or sleep terror episodes if they are genetically predisposed to them.

- **Autistic children** (and others with different neuropsychiatric developmental disorders) are particularly prone to sleep problems the origins of which are again likely to be a mixture of behavioural and physical factors. The behavioural sleep problems of autistic children respond to the same behavioural treatments that are effective in other children, but sleep disturbance due to other influences (such as an underlying medical condition) require an additional, different approach.

- **Other psychiatric conditions** in which sleep disturbance can be particularly prominent include conduct disorders (in which difficult and possibly ill-disciplined behaviour can affect sleep habits), obsessive–compulsive behaviour, eating disorders, and alcohol or other substance misuse.

- The effects of some **psychotropic medications** used to treat behavioural and psychiatric conditions can affect sleep patterns adversely. Some antidepressants can cause difficulties in sleeping, even though they help to relieve the depression. As mentioned in connection with ADHD, the drugs given for this condition may disturb sleep because of their stimulant properties. Sedative or tranquillizing drugs can make you sleepy during the day.

📄 Case study

Autism

A 5-year-old boy was considered to have classical signs of autism with impaired relationships with other people (including his parents), odd use of language and other means of communication, and strange ritualistic behaviour, as well as unusual mannerisms. These features had begun to show themselves from the age of 2.

In common with many other autistic children, he had always been difficult to get to sleep at bedtime. He awoke repeatedly at night, insisting on attention from his parents, and he often woke up early in the morning and could not get back to sleep, causing much commotion.

Sleeping medicines had failed to be effective and his parents were at a loss as to what to do next. Although they had read about behavioural treatments for sleepless children in general, they did not think that they could be used with an autistic child such as their son because of his communication difficulties, his characteristic resistance to change, and his generally high anxiety levels.

However, because the situation was becoming so fraught, their local clinical psychologist thought it was worth a try and, with her support, they embarked on a well worked out behavioural treatment programme (see Chapter 5). Over the first few days, the boy became more upset than ever at night, but, with encouragement, his parents persisted and by the next month he was settling to sleep at bedtime and then sleeping quite soundly during the night. Only sometimes was his early morning waking a problem, but his relieved parents were prepared to put up with this.

21

Misinterpretation of children's sleep disorders

➡ Key points

◆ It is important to recognize sleep disorders for what they really are and not mistake them for other conditions.

◆ Failure to recognize sleep disorders can mean failure to provide the correct advice or treatment for a child's condition, which may well result in upset and frustration for both the child and his family.

◆ As it is possible for a child to have more than one sleep disorder (or a sleep disorder and also some other type of problem), careful assessment of a child's overall condition is essential.

✖ Myth versus fact

Myth: It is obvious if someone has a sleep disorder.

Fact: This is definitely not always the case. As knowledge about the nature and likely effects of disordered sleep is often lacking, there seem to be many instances of sleep disorders and their consequences being misinterpreted, overlooked, or ignored completely. This is likely to have serious consequences.

At a number of places in this book, reference has been made to the risk that sleep disorders of various types may be mistaken for other, very different types of condition. If this happens, the consequences could be serious in that the wrong kind of advice or treatment will be given. It is appropriate to say something more about this problem.

Professional advice is sought in only the minority of children and adolescents with a significant sleep problem. Lack of awareness by parents that is—in principle—possible is probably the main explanation for this, but failure to realise that a child's behaviour is the result of sleep difficulties is also likely to be a factor. That being so, the following points about possible misinterpretations are worth emphasizing.

The prospect of sleep disorders being misinterpreted as other psychological or medical conditions is increased when the parents themselves, or relatives and friends giving advice, or the professionals whom they consult for help simply do not know enough about the many types of sleep disturbance or the various ways in which they can affect your child. The limited knowledge about such matters is no surprise in view of the low level of attention paid to sleep and its disorders in public health education, parenting classes, and professional training.

The general point is that, if your child persistently does not get enough sleep or the quality of his sleep is poor, then the way he feels and behaves is likely to be affected in a number of unwelcome ways (see Chapter 2). Tiredness, irritability, poor concentration, impaired performance at school or college, and depression are common examples of this.

Excessive daytime sleepiness, whatever its cause (see the many possibilities mentioned in Chapter 8), is often misjudged as laziness, disinterest and daydreaming, lack of motivation, depression, intellectual inadequacy, or a number of other states of mind. A sleep disorder may be the starting point for the troublesome daytime behaviour in some children with attention-deficit hyperactivity disorder (ADHD).

📄 Case study

Disturbed sleep misdiagnosed as ADHD

A health visitor was asked by her GP colleague to advise on a 4-year-old boy whose behaviour was very disturbed both at home (including sleeping very badly) and at school where he was very disruptive. From what they had seen on a television programme, his parents had come to believe that he had ADHD, which they thought should be treated with drugs to calm him down.

The GP was aware that the term ADHD is sometimes used for children with various problems for which different types of advice and treatment are required. For example, some are overactive and difficult to control because they have not learned to behave properly, whilst others are restless and cannot concentrate at school because they are anxious or bored there. Sometimes, on careful enquiry, the child's behaviour is actually found to be appropriate for his age but his parents cannot cope with it because they themselves are emotionally upset or depressed. It was hoped that the health visitor's enquiries could help decide what the situation really was in this case.

Her thorough assessment included looking into the boy's sleep patterns and anything that might affect them. It came to light that, as part of a generally disorganized home life, he had for some time been in the habit of drinking up to six cans of a cola drink most days, and each night went to bed very late with a large bottle of milky coffee. Needless to say, his daily intake of caffeine was extremely high and was disrupting his sleep.

It was apparent that the boy's ADHD-type behaviour was largely the result of a combination of a chaotic way of life, a high-caffeine intake and inadequate sleep. Unfortunately, attempts to correct these influences were only partly successful and the boy's behaviour remained a problem.

Treatment with the type of drugs often used for ADHD due to genuine neurodevelopmental factors would have been inappropriate in this situation, and there would have been a risk that they could have added to the boy's sleeping problems.

Specific sleep disorders

The features of many individual sleep disorders are open to misinterpretations of a more specific nature. Some examples of this in children and adolescents in general are given below.

A common cause of confusion and mistakes is the tendency to use the term **nightmare** for any dramatic parasomnia of which there are, in fact, many types. The correct meaning of nightmare is given in Chapter 16.

Generally, it is not realized that complicated behaviour can occur while someone remains asleep during the quite common arousal disorders such as **sleepwalking** (see Chapter 15). Although some sleepwalking episodes involve fairly calm walking about in a semi-purposeful (although often accident-prone) way, some sleepwalkers do much more complicated things such as making drinks or meals, wandering outside the house, and even driving a car.

Children with agitated sleepwalking or **sleep terrors** appear to be very fearful or distressed and to rush about and cry out as if escaping from danger. Some people develop an eating disorder with excessive weight gain due to the amount of food they consume while they are still asleep at night. Rarely, sleepwalkers behave in an aggressive or destructive way, causing injury to themselves or others, and (at least in adults) sexual offences have sometimes been committed in the course of a sleepwalking episode.

Clearly, if it is not known that such complicated behaviours are compatible with still being asleep, it will be assumed that the person was awake at the time and aware of what they were doing, and that they are therefore responsible for what happened.

The difficulties in getting to sleep and also waking in the morning, as well as daytime sleepiness and sleeping in at the weekend, that characterize **delayed sleep-phase syndrome** (DSPS) (see Chapters 7 and 9) are easily misinterpreted as awkward, lazy, or irresponsible behaviour, malingering, or refusal to go to school, especially in adolescents in whom DSPS is common. In fact, this sleep disorder is the result of a combination of biological body clock and lifestyle changes. The risk of the fundamental problem not being recognized is increased if alcohol or sedative drugs are taken in an attempt to get to sleep, or stimulants are used to try and stay awake during the day.

Other gross disturbances of sleep–wake patterns can occur with **abuse of alcohol and other substances**, causing profound psychological effects that might not be the result of disrupted sleep.

Obstructive sleep apnoea (see Chapter 10) in children can cause excessive sleepiness and reduced activity, but can also cause the opposite effect, i.e. overactivity and other troublesome behaviour, as well as learning problems. Correction of the breathing difficulty at night can be expected to improve daytime behaviour and learning, which otherwise are likely be attributed to other, very different causes.

Narcolepsy (see Chapter 11) is another example of how sleepiness can be misinterpreted. When (as is usual) cataplexy is also present, there is even more scope for such mistakes. At all ages, many years often elapse before these conditions are correctly recognized. In the meantime, sufferers are likely to be treated for various psychological states (including, in the case of children, misbehaviour or attention-seeking behaviour) or other physical conditions such as fainting attacks or epilepsy. It is likely that some cases of narcolepsy/cataplexy are never correctly recognized.

Parents of the many young children with **rhythmic movement disorder** (see Chapter 13) may mistakenly think that this is because of an emotional problem or is perhaps some form of epilepsy. Parents and children can also be reassured about the common experiences of **isolated sleep paralysis** (i.e. other than that associated with narcolepsy), which might be thought to be a neurological disorder, or **sleep-related hallucinations** (see Chapter 13), which, in their most dramatic form (especially if combined with sleep paralysis), may be thought to be part of a mental disorder.

A number of other sleep-related conditions, although individually not particularly common, are also often not correctly recognized, with potentially serious consequences. The particularly severe and episodic sleepiness in the **Kleine–Levin syndrome** (see Chapter 11) in which, when the person is awake, they often demonstrate strange and out-of-character behaviour, understandably causes confusion in the minds of those who are unfamiliar with the condition. Some people with this condition, including older children and adolescents, may initially be thought to have a serious brain disease, drug-abuse problems, or a psychiatric illness.

Similarly, the violent behaviour during sleep displayed by those (including some children) with the **REM sleep behaviour disorder** (RBD) (see Chapter 16) when acting out their dreams is likely to be misconstrued as some other condition including another type of parasomnia.

The form of sleep-related epilepsy known as **nocturnal frontal lobe epilepsy** (see Chapter 18) also often involves seizures that include dramatic movements and noises. As these episodes are most unlike other types of epileptic seizure, it may well be thought that the condition is not epilepsy at all but something quite different, such as a psychological disorder or even that the person is pretending to have epilepsy.

📄 Case study

Epilepsy misdiagnosed as 'nightmares' and 'pseudoseizures'

For about the last 2 years, a 12-year-old girl had been having strange episodes, mainly at night, in which she suddenly stopped what she was doing, or woke up, seeming to be vague and out of touch with her surroundings.

She would then start bouncing about either round the room or on the top of her bed, making grunting noises in time with the movements.

Although these incidents occurred infrequently during the day, they caused some consternation to her parents and teachers, although her classmates tended to think them amusing. Her parents became even more concerned when the episodes began to happen up to eight times a night at various times.

Each episode lasted no more the about half a minute at the end of which time, during the day, she would suddenly became her usual self again. At night, she promptly went back to sleep as soon as the episode was over. She only knew what had happened if she was told about the episode afterwards.

In other respects, she was perfectly healthy, as she had been all her life. She was popular and intelligent, was doing well at school and did not have any emotional problems. Despite this, because they were so peculiar, her daytime episodes were initially thought to be attention-seeking behaviour—pretend seizures or 'pseudoseizures'. Those occurring at night were labelled 'nightmares', even though she remained asleep throughout them with no description of any frightening dreams. Her parents were not happy with these diagnoses and pressed for her to be referred to a paediatric neurologist who was known to have a special interest in sleep disorders.

As the episodes were so frequent, it was possible to record an electroen-cephalogram during some of them, both during the day and at night. This clearly showed that each episode was accompanied by epileptic discharges starting in the front part of the brain on one side. These findings confirmed the suspicion of the neurologist that the girl had the form of epilepsy known as 'nocturnal frontal lobe epilepsy' (in which some of the seizures can occur during the day, although they mainly occur at night during sleep). The diagnoses of 'nightmares' and 'pseudoseizures' had been completely wrong.

Further investigations showed no sign of any serious underlying cause of her epilepsy and she responded well to treatment with anti-epileptic medication.

In considering all these possible ways in which sleep disorders may not be recognized for what they really are, it is, of course, important to recognize that your child may have a combination of a sleep disorder and other conditions of a different nature—or, indeed, more than one type of sleep disorder. **Parasomnia overlap disorder** is an admittedly unusual example of a combination of different parasomnias. In this sleep disorder, people of various ages (including children and adolescents) have a combination of sleepwalking, sleep terrors, and RBD, sometimes associated with physical or psychiatric disorders.

This and other examples make it all the more important that, as described towards the beginning of the book, each sleep problem and its cause is assessed thoroughly by someone familiar with the range of possible explanations. Without this, there is a serious risk that a wrong conclusion will be reached. This is likely to cause you and your child unnecessary concern and also to deny your child the correct and probably effective treatment for his sleep disorder.

22

Being vigilant

➡ Key point

◆ Many sleep disorders are misinterpreted or overlooked; therefore, a combined effort is needed on the part of children themselves (if old enough), parents, teachers, and other professionals to recognize unsatisfactory sleep in order for its harmful effects to be prevented.

✖ Myth versus fact

Myth: Sleep problems are mainly a private matter that other people cannot really help with.

Fact: If the effects of disturbed sleep are known, they can be recognized, leading to the provision of effective treatment.

Reference has been made previously to the fact that knowledge about sleep problems, their causes, and their treatment is often lacking, both in the general population and among various professional groups.

A major consequence of this is that, as highlighted in Chapter 21, many treatable sleep disorders are misconstrued or even ignored, even though their consequences can be serious and, in the case of children, harmful to their psychological, educational, and sometimes physical development. Relatively few receive the help that could be made available to the benefit of the children themselves and also their families.

It is no exaggeration, as has been said (particularly in the USA), that the neglect of sleep disorders and their effects is a major public health issue. Better health education about such matters is required all round, but, although awareness is improving somewhat, progress is slow and much more needs to be achieved. In the meantime, encouragement can be given to those involved in the health and welfare of children to be more vigilant and sensitive to sleep problems, their possible causes, and how they might be prevented or treated.

Prevention or treatment of the harmful effects of not having enough sleep on learning, behaviour, and social relationships ideally calls for a co-ordinated effort on the part of older children themselves (especially teenagers), as well as their parents, teachers, and other professionals.

Children and teenagers

There are good reasons for including sleep in the school curriculum along side other biological and health-related subjects. Certainly, teenagers need to be aware of the significance of persistently having problems getting to sleep, of waking frequently in the night, or having great difficulty getting up in the morning. This is especially so if they are tired or actually falling asleep during the day, feel slowed down, irritable, or depressed, and perhaps have mood swings, as well as difficulty concentrating, remembering things, or making decisions properly. Sleeping in very late at weekends is another warning sign that they are not getting enough sleep and that they have built up what is called a 'sleep debt'.

Parents

It seems that parents often do not know about teenagers' sleep problems. They should suspect such problems if it is particularly difficult to rouse their child in the morning, or if he falls asleep doing homework, needs caffeine drinks, or sleeps very late at weekends. It is obviously significant if his behaviour is better after a good night's sleep or if a teacher has mentioned tiredness during the day as a problem (see Chapter 2).

Teachers

Teachers themselves should consider a sleep problem as a possible explanation of difficulties at school, for example if a child's school performance levels decrease or if there is a change in behaviour taking the form of poor concentration, little energy, a lack of motivation, withdrawal, nervousness, difficult behaviour, or missing or being late for school.

Other professionals

Sleep problems in young people are very common and their effects are diverse. As a result, because of the misinterpretations already discussed in Chapter 21, children may be referred inappropriately to services that concern themselves with the effects of the sleep disorder without realizing their real cause.

For example, child and adolescent psychiatrists and child psychologists are asked to advise on disturbed behaviour for which various possible traditional explanations will readily be considered. The effects of inadequate or disturbed sleep should be added to these explanations. The same is true of some referrals to educational psychologists for poor progress at school and, indeed, those to paediatricians for various physical complaints.

Advice for young people

Advice about sleep can very reasonably be seen as a fundamental part of health education, especially for adolescents. Points of special emphasis are that young people of this age should aim for at least 9 hours of sleep at night. As discussed before, good sleep hygiene means avoiding irregular sleep patterns, too much caffeine (in coffee, cola, and stimulant drinks), exciting and prolonged activities at bedtime (in the form of TV or computer use, phone calls, and texting), and heavy meals and vigorous exercise in the late evening.

Lying in bed awake for long periods sets up the unhelpful link between bed and being awake instead of being ready to sleep. Sleeping in until very late at weekends confuses the body clock and maintains the abnormal sleep pattern on weekdays. An unhealthy diet, too little exercise, smoking, and immoderate amounts of alcohol are also capable of disturbing sleep in their different ways. It is best for children and adolescents with a sleep problem to tell their parents so that the solution can be found jointly.

These are examples of relatively straightforward help and advice that can be provided for young people, but, for this to happen, it is clearly necessary for all involved in their care and welfare to be vigilant and also well informed about the importance of satisfactory sleep.

23

Getting help with your child's sleep problem

➡ **Key points**

◆ The help needed for your child's sleep problem, and who might provide it, depends on how complicated the problem is.

◆ The sequence of possible steps in obtaining help can be: self-help (only useful up to a point); consulting your GP or health visitor; seeing a hospital specialist; and attending a sleep disorders clinic.

◆ Precise diagnosis should lead to effective treatment if carried out properly.

❌ **Myth versus fact**

Myth: No help is available for sleep problems—you just have to put up with them.

Fact: Although there is room for improvement in the provision of help with sleep problems, many effective treatments of different types have been developed and can be made available if the right avenues are explored.

The point has been made repeatedly throughout this book that, because disturbed sleep can compromise a child's development and general well-being in a variety of ways, it is very important that sleep problems should be prevented where possible or treated effectively if already established. The key to achieving this is accurate diagnosis of the underlying cause of your child's sleep problem. How can this be secured?

Self-help

This really means parents recognizing the signs that their child's sleep is unsatisfactory and finding out what can be done to improve matters (see Chapter 2). Clearly, this has to be the responsibility of parents of young children, but adolescents themselves may be capable of doing this to some extent.

The first step is to learn more about sleep and its disorders, given that, as mentioned elsewhere, it is a generally neglected topic. Reading about such things in this book or from other sources will help to provide at least a background knowledge.

Even just observing the sleep hygiene principles also discussed in Chapter 2, or trying the effect of the measures suggested in subsequent chapters depending on the age of your child, may be helpful. This is certainly preferable to relying on over-the-counter products from a chemist or health food shop without the real nature of the problem being established.

Professional help

As well as self-help, seeking professional advice is often advisable and should be sought if your own efforts have been unsuccessful, if the nature of the underlying cause of your child's sleep problem is unclear, if you are confused from your reading about what should be done, or if you or your child are worried or distressed about the problem.

Your first port of call should be your family doctor or, for a very young child, your health visitor. Your doctor can at least make a start in assessing the nature of your child's problem and may well be able to suggest appropriate treatment (this is rarely medication).

In some localities, health visitors provide a special skilled service for tackling the sleep problems of babies and young children, including organizing group instruction for parents.

Depending on the initial findings, and to explore further possible medical or psychological factors, your doctor may suggest that you take your child to see a specialist, for example a paediatrician if there is a possibility that your child has a breathing problem at night (such as obstructive sleep apnoea), or a child psychologist or psychiatrist if help with an emotional problem seems to be needed.

Sleep disorders clinics

If the explanation for your child's sleep problem remains unclear, or seems particularly complicated or difficult to treat, it is advisable for your doctor to refer him to a specialized sleep disorders clinic, preferably where there is special interest in children's sleep disorders. Here, you can expect the more detailed assessments described in Chapter 2, including sleep studies, where appropriate. On the basis of an accurate diagnosis, treatment can then be recommended and its effectiveness evaluated, usually by the clinic staff in conjunction with your GP or other local services.

Children can sometimes be seen privately by staff working in NHS units. Otherwise, there are a few private sleep clinics.

Outlook

If advice and treatment for your child's sleep problem is based on careful assessment of the cause of his problem, and if it is followed in detail and with persistence (which may require professional supervision and support in difficult cases), the outcome is likely to be good.

If your child's sleep can be improved, his prospects will be better and the quality of your own life will also be improved.

Appendix

Relevant organizations

British Sleep Society
PO Box 247
Colne
Huntington PE28 3 UZ
Email: enquiries@sleeping.org.uk
Website: www.sleeping.org.uk

SleepScotland
8 Hope Park Square
Edinburgh EH8 9NW
Website: www.sleepscotland.org

Further reading

Stores, G. (2001) *A Clinical Guide to Sleep Disorders in Children and Adolescents.* Cambridge: Cambridge University Press.

Stores, G. (2009) *Insomnia and Other Adult Sleep Problems: The Facts.* Oxford: Oxford University Press.

Stores, G, Wiggs, L. (eds) (2001) *Sleep Disturbance in Children and Adolescents with Disorders of Development: its Significance and Management.* London: Mac Keith Press.

Glossary

The following are some basic terms used in this book. Other definitions are provided in the text.

Active sleep: equivalent in infants to REM sleep.

Actometry (actigraphy): technique by which a wristwatch-like device is used to measure body movements to help distinguish between periods of sleep and wakefulness.

Advanced sleep phase: shift of the period of sleep to earlier than usual in the 24-hour sleep–wake cycle.

Audio-visual recordings: mainly recordings (including home recordings by parents) to show a child's condition and any events overnight. Can be particularly valuable in describing parasomnias and in obstructive sleep apnoea.

Apnoea: interruption of breathing (technically for a minimum of about 10 seconds).

Arousal disorders: sleep disorders (confusional arousals, sleepwalking, and sleep terrors) that emerge abruptly from deep NREM sleep.

Cataplexy: sudden weakness provoked by strong emotions such as laughter, surprise, fear, or anger. Can cause a collapse or localized weakness lasting from a few seconds to minutes without loss of consciousness and with prompt recovery.

Chronic fatigue syndrome or **CFS** (also known as **myalgic encephalomyelitis** or **ME**): persistent or episodic fatigue and muscle pain of uncertain cause that does not lessen with sleep or rest.

Circadian rhythm: rhythm, including the sleep–wake cycle, that occurs about once every 24 hours, generally tied to the 24-hour night–day cycle.

Comfort (or transitional) object: object, such as a favourite toy or piece of blanket, that helps a child to feel secure and accept the separation from his parents at night.

Conditioned insomnia: difficulty sleeping, the original cause of which no longer operates but which has led to habitual insomnia by association.

Delayed sleep phase: shift of the sleep phase to later than usual in the 24-hour sleep–wake cycle.

Early morning waking: in general, waking up before about 5 a.m. and not being able to go back to sleep.

Electroencephalogram (EEG): recording of the electrical activity of the brain by means of electrodes placed on the scalp. Combined with an electro-myogram and electro-oculogram, an EEG allows scoring of the sleep stages and waking.

Electromyogram (EMG): recording of the electrical activity of muscles; for sleep studies, the activity of the chin muscles is recorded.

Electro-oculogram (EOG): recording of eye movements using electrodes placed on the face.

Excessive daytime sleepiness or hypersomnia: increased tendency or need to fall asleep.

Hypnagogic hallucinations or imagery: vivid perceptual experiences involving various senses when going to sleep.

Hypnogram: diagram of the structure of overnight sleep showing the sequence of sleep stages and periods of waking.

Hypnopompic hallucinations or imagery: unusual perceptual experiences when waking up.

Hypocretin (orexin): neurotransmitter in the brain involved in the control of sleep. Low levels are found in people with narcolepsy/cataplexy.

Multiple sleep latency test (MSLT): objective test of sleepiness in which the opportunity to fall asleep is given four or five times during the day. The time taken to fall asleep each time, and the stage of sleep near the start of sleep, can help in the diagnosis of narcolepsy in particular.

Nap: short period of sleep taken during the day. Normal in young children.

Nightmare: frightening dream, arising in REM sleep (and therefore usually late in the night), that causes awakening.

Non-rapid eye movement (NREM) sleep: one of the two basic types of sleep, distinct from rapid eye movement (REM) sleep. Divided into four stages of increasing depth of sleep.

Parasomnia: episode of unusual behaviour or a strange experience related to sleep.

Periodic limb movements in sleep (PLMS): repetitive, brief, rapid flexion movements, mainly in the legs, during sleep.

Polysomnogram (PSG): continuous recording of sleep by means of an EEG, EMG and EOG, with the possible addition of breathing or other physiological measures depending on the nature of the sleep problem.

Quiet sleep: equivalent in infants of NREM sleep.

Rapid eye movement (REM) sleep: type of sleep with the highest brain activity. Also known as 'dreaming sleep' because most dreaming occurs in it, and also 'paradoxical sleep' because, although brain activity is high, the skeletal muscles are effectively paralysed.

Seasonal affective disorder (SAD): daytime fatigue and sleepiness, poor concentration, and increased appetite and weight gain, mainly in the winter months.

Sleep diary: daily written record of a person's sleep–wake pattern and related events.

Sleep disorder: underlying condition causing a sleep problem.

Sleep hygiene: ways of improving sleep or preventing poor sleep. Useful in its own right but can be helpful combined with more specific treatment for a sleep disorder.

Sleeplessness: difficulty getting to sleep or staying asleep. Equivalent to 'insomnia' in older children and adults.

Sleep paralysis: brief inability to move or speak when falling asleep or waking up. May be accompanied by a feeling of an inability to breathe and by hypnagogic hallucinations. Can be very frightening. Common as an isolated experience but can be part of the narcolepsy syndrome.

Sleep problem: complaint of disturbed or abnormal sleep.

Sleep start: sudden brief movement or sensory experience (possibly alarming) when going off to sleep.

Sleep–wake cycle: alternation of sleep and wakefulness in each 24-hour period.

Slow wave sleep (SWS): the combination of stages 3 and 4 of NREM sleep, the deepest parts of sleep. Also called 'delta sleep' referring to the large, slow (delta) waves that predominate.

Snoring: noise (which can be considerable) produced by a large intake of breath at the end of an apnoea or partial apnoea. Due to vibration of the soft palate and nearby structures.

Zeitgeber: literally a 'time giver' that informs the brain whether it is day or night, and which therefore indicates whether it is time to be awake or asleep.

Index